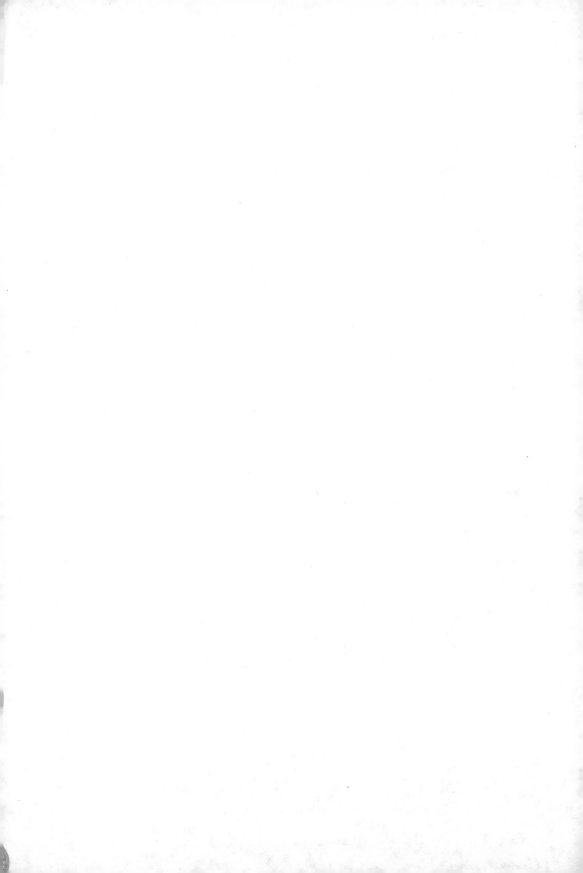

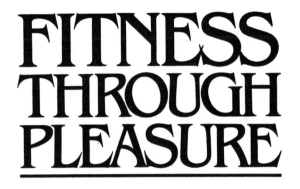

FITNESS THROUGH PLEASURE

Editor: Bill Gottlieb

Research Chief: Carol Baldwin
Research Coordinator: Sue Ann Gursky
Research Associates:
  Carol Matthews
  Martha Capwell
  Trieste Kennedy
  Christy Kohler
  Susan Nastasee
  Susan Rosenkrantz

Copy Editor: Barbara Nykoruk

Assistant Editor: Marian Wolbers

Library:
  Liz Wolbach
  Colleen Garis

Office Personnel:
  Diana Gottshall
  Barbara Hill
  Sue Lagler
  Brenda Peluso
  Carol Petrakovich
  Donna Strubeck

Executive Fitness Newsletter
  Associate Editor: Heidi Rodale

Executive Fitness Newsletter
  Research Director: Mark Schwartz, Ph.D.

Executive Fitness Newsletter
  Readers' Service: Janice Saad

FITNESS THROUGH PLEASURE

A GUIDE TO SUPERIOR HEALTH
for people who like to have a good time

Porter Shimer
Executive Editor,
Executive Fitness Newsletter®

Rodale Press, Emmaus, Pa.

Book Design: Merole Berger
Book Layout: John Pepper

Printed in the United States of America on recycled paper, containing a high
percentage of de-inked fiber.

Library of Congress Cataloging in Publication Data

Shimer, Porter.
    Fitness through pleasure.

    Includes index.
    1. Physical fitness. 2. Health. 3. Nutrition.
I. Title.
GV481.S476   613.7'1   82–5430
ISBN 0–87857–398–4 hardcover   AACR2

2   4   6   8   10   9   7   5   3   hardcover

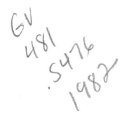
I dedicate this book to Mark Bricklin for finding, teaching, provoking, inspiring, and enduring me. And special thanks to my wife, Connie, who can recite this book by heart.

ACKNOWLEDGMENTS

Whether anybody's ever said it before or not, somebody should have: "If you've got something you want heard, make it short."

Thank you, Bill Gottlieb, Sue Ann Gursky, Marian Wolbers, Diana Gottshall, Sue Lagler, Carol Petrakovich, Barbara Hill, Brenda Peluso, Janice Saad, Carl Sherman, Jean Rogers, Judi Davenport, Liz Wolbach, and Ethel Bloss. You all know who you are.

FOREWORD

In looking at the health field in the United States and other industrial nations, it's clear that most of our health problems are not caused by the infectious diseases that just a few decades ago were the major killers. Today, plagues and epidemics aren't much of a threat—*but stress is.* Headaches, arthritis, low back pain, heart attacks, strokes—these are some of the stress-related disorders that "plague" modern man. This modern plague isn't going to be eradicated by new drugs and vaccines. It will take preventive action to stop diseases caused by stress. And the most important factor in prevention is *you.*

Only you can stop dangerous health habits like smoking, overeating, overdrinking, and lack of exercise. These types of habits increase your risk for all kinds of stress-related problems. But it's not only what we do habitually to the body that makes us ill. It's also what we do with our mental attitudes—particularly the hard-driving, hostile, and impatient attitude characteristic of the Type A personality—which increases our susceptibility to disease. A heart attack, for instance, is 250 percent more likely among Type A individuals.

We don't have to wait until a heart attack to learn the habits of good health. We should set up personal programs—now—to develop healthier habits of body and mind. I have worked in this field of developing health and stress-management programs in hospital, industrial, and community settings. For instance, in my capacity as Chief of Biofeedback Service at Saint Luke's–Roosevelt Hospital in New York City, I have helped implement programs in behavior modification and biofeedback in the treatment of obesity, high blood pressure, headaches, and other stress-related disorders. I have learned that—even with medicine in the United States offering some of the most highly technical and competent solutions for these health problems—the first step toward well-being of body and mind is a personal preventive program.

In this book, *Fitness through Pleasure,* Porter Shimer offers just such a program to take better care of yourself. He offers, first, an underlying philosophy of "moderation." Instead of a punishing fitness program (or an unrealistically easy one), he outlines how to gain fitness by making use of your personal need for pleasure and happiness. In fact, he tells you how to change habits *without* taking the enjoyment out of life, and his idea of "fitness through pleasure" is one that can work for everyone.

Further, this book will give useful hints and specific information on how to design a personal program of physical exercise, good diet, and healthy attitude. These suggestions can be used by the executive, the housewife, or anyone who is willing to learn how to take better care of his or her body and mind.

I urge you to read and use this book rather than waiting and hoping that you will not get a stress-related disease or disorder. You can, by putting into practice the "pleasure principle" behind fitness and health, become more energetic and happier. Remember, it's not inevitable that you experience stress-related problems. Let us all work together to experience better health, and then we can all work to make the world a more enjoyable and pleasurable place to live. *Fitness through Pleasure* will help you make health a reality. Read it and put it to use!

Keith Sedlacek, M.D.
Chief of Biofeedback Service
Investigator in Biofeedback and Stress-Related Disorders
Department of Psychiatry
Saint Luke's–Roosevelt Hospital
Faculty—Columbia Medical School

CONTENTS

LIST OF TABLES

PROLOGUE

When I was about nine, I made a parachute out of a bed sheet and some clothesline and went into a field behind our house during a windstorm for the express purpose of getting knocked down and dragged around by Mother Nature. It was fun. But as I recall, it was also quite a workout.

Etched in grass stains on that bed sheet were the beginnings of an unusual career in physical fitness and, more importantly, a principle that would eventually become the kingpin of the *Executive Fitness Newsletter*.

That principle?

That the pursuit of health can be fun; and that it should be. We live with enough stress as it is. We don't need burdensome health routines to weigh on us even more.

INTRODUCTION

Where Happiness Goes, Health Follows

We all know someone who has managed to live long and live well despite breaking a considerable number of what health professionals tell us are the rules. (I have a great aunt, age 79, who drinks beer and smokes unfiltered cigarettes. She even swears more than she should.)

How do these people do it?

Certainly a strong genetic background helps. And often these people will have good habits that tend to get overshadowed by their bad ones. (My great aunt, when she's not smoking or swearing, eats a lot of vegetables.)

It's the premise of this book, however, that something else is at play. And that something else is pleasure.

Several years ago an interesting study was reported in the *New England Journal of Medicine* (December 6, 1979) by George E. Vaillant, an M.D. from Cambridge Hospital. Dr. Vaillant kept track of the lives of 188 male graduates of Harvard University for a period of 32 years. From the time these men enrolled at Harvard until the time they reached their early fifties in 1975, he kept records of their physical and mental health. What Dr. Vaillant was looking for was a connection between the two. And he found one.

The men whose lives had been emotionally stable reported less than half the physical illnesses than did the men whose lives had been emotionally rocky. Their happiness, in fact, proved to be a more reliable indicator of good health than how much the men smoked, drank, or were overweight.

Then there was the rabbit study done at the University of Houston. Scientists investigating heart disease discovered by accident that rabbits could be made significantly more resistant to the ill effects of a high-cholesterol diet when taken from their cages and subjected to regular daily pettings (*Science*, June, 1980).

The moral of these stories?

That life is easier to live when it feels good. When we're happy—or unhappy—every cell in our bodies gets the message.

The notion of mind and body being in close communication is not new. The Greeks were on to the idea two thousand years ago. But over the past few centuries, in preference to approaches that treated the body *or* the mind, the concept got put aside. It's back in the limelight, though, and showing brighter promise than ever. As Dr. Vaillant was prompted to remark regarding the

Harvard study, "Instead of just some illnesses being psychosomatic, there is now evidence that psychosocial factors play a role in *all* illnesses."

Our health, in other words, appears to be largely in our heads. There is a "will to live," after all. It has the ability to bring about specific and measurable biological events. And, luckily, it seems to have a very good friend in pleasure.

Before you make off to the kitchen to buddy up to another double scotch, however, understand that science is also discovering that pleasure is most healthfully pursued for the right reasons, and with restraint. Pleasurable pursuits in moderation can refurbish, but in excess they can delude and destroy.

Which brings us to the purpose of this book. We're not going to try to get you to *quit* anything, or even cut down if you decide you really don't want to. Because health, as noted psychologist Kenneth R. Pelletier, Ph.D., has said, is a matter of "following little messages from inside that tell you what's right for you, no matter what some 'expert' might say."

But then you won't find us recommending lost weekends in Las Vegas, either. It's our firm belief that moderation is the highest way to fly because it entices the senses instead of numbing them, as abuse does. What we hope to do in the following pages is to sharpen your appetite for pleasure so that you will be better able to experience it in forms—and in amounts—that are good for you.

And how do we propose to do that?

By improving your health. The purer you get your body, the less it takes to show it a good time. And a better time it will have. A case in point . . .

When I was in my invincible twenties, I would go to some very unusual lengths to exhaust myself. My efforts earned me a resting pulse of 35 and a physique about as padded as a park bench. I went overboard, granted, but sometimes it takes going overboard to get a better look at the ship.

What I learned from my experiences was that the body is a sucker for contrasts. Two beers would be as satisfying as four after my workouts in the summer. And sitting by a wood stove would feel like sitting in the Oval Office after my ordeals in the winter. I was very fit and so, I'm convinced, very sensitive to whatever I would do to give myself pleasure.

I am in no way suggesting unmitigated pain for you joggers. What I am suggesting, though, is jogging shoes for you sedentaries. And perhaps a touch of Spartanism for you Romans. By sharpening ourselves physically, we sharpen our appetites for food, drink, relaxation, sex . . . the joys of life in general.

If the above story has you thinking that this book might not be for you, relax. There's something here for everybody. If a pulse of 35 is the last thing on your mind, and all you want is to keep whatever it is you're currently doing for pleasure from killing you, pay attention to part 1 of this book.

But if the prospect of superior health *does* intrigue you (and trust us, it's easier than you might think), then pay attention to part 2. Whichever route you choose, however, keep one thing in mind: "If it feels good, it can't be all bad."

At the risk of leading some of the weaker-willed among us down paths of total ruin, I honestly believe that's true. Conventional health propaganda seems to overlook the fact that we all have our darker moments; that we can be frustrated, self-doubting, and depressed; and that we each have our own best ways of working such moods out, however contrary to accepted health wisdom those ways may be. Which does not mean, however, that they are wrong. What impressed Dr. Vaillant most about the men who were healthiest in his study was not so much their physical lifestyles as it was the "hierarchy of defense mechanisms" by which each handled life's ups and downs *as he saw fit.* Indeed, the individuality factor is one that the medical profession seems to have slighted.

You, potentially, are your best doctor. Learn from this book the basics of health, then adapt them to *your* needs. We increase our chances of living to be 100 as much by doing what we can to be *happy* as by doing what we can to be healthy. And who, better than you, can say what makes you happy?

To your health,
Porter Shimer

PART I/
HOW TO KEEP
BAD HABITS
FROM KILLING YOU

Our Need for Pleasure Is in Our Genes

Those of us who can't seem to stay on diets or get much of a rise out of doing push-ups would do well to look back a few thousand years. Neither diets nor push-ups played much of a role in our evolutionary development. Anybody caught doing a push-up ten thousand years ago, in fact, might have been thought of as having a problem. And anybody substantially reducing his caloric intake would have died. Crash diets and distasteful exercise routines are modern-day medicines for modern-day ills. The reason they're so hard to swallow is that they run counter to our survivalistic instincts.

No, the way to health in the old days was not through pain but through pleasure—pleasure in eating, securing shelter, and having sex. Things worked out so that what felt good was also good for us. Then we complicated matters.

We discovered alcohol, tobacco, drugs, fast cars, and cheesecake—all of which have the potential for affording us pleasure *without* being good for us. At the heart of our modern-day health problems, quite simply, is the fact that we are pleasure-seeking creatures now being asked to survive amidst pleasures that are not always healthful to seek. An estimated 34 percent of us smoke, 68 percent drink, and 25 percent are overweight. But not because we're suicidal —just the opposite is true. We're looking to get out of life all the pleasure we can, which is basically a very healthful urge. Because pleasure nourishes optimism. And of all our longevity factors, optimism may be one of the most crucial.

As noted author and anthropologist Lionel Tiger points out, optimism helped keep us alive as cave people, and it can help keep us alive today. There was a distinct advantage to be gained by the cave person capable of remaining optimistic in the face of adversity, so optimism as a human trait got passed along. And methods for keeping optimism alive got passed along, too: religion, holidays, chocolate chip cookies, alcohol. Anything that lifts our spirits has potential for helping us survive. Which is why we make ourselves a drink to lift our spirits after a lousy day at work. We're giving in to the urge to keep our chins up, an urge that has been thousands of years in the making.

Optimism, however, isn't the only thing we're trying to keep alive when we reach for the likes of our liquor bottles. There's our sense of justice. Whenever we experience displeasure we feel the need for some pleasure to balance that displeasure out. When our stomachs signal that they're being short-changed, for example, we go for lunch.

On a more emotional level, however, our sense of justice can make us curse in traffic jams, smoke when we're nervous, or overeat when we're depressed. Somewhere in our brains, our pleasure-stats are saying, "You've experienced displeasure; you need pleasure to balance that displeasure out. If you do not get it, you will not be happy—and, as a result, you may decrease your chances of remaining *optimistic* enough to survive."

If all of this sounds a little too philosophical, reflect for a moment on the following real-life scenarios.

- You've moved all of two car lengths on the freeway in a matter of half an hour. So when things finally get rolling, you pull off onto the first side road you can find and floor it—not to make up for lost time so much as to make up for acquired misery.

Simply a release of frustration, you say?

Well, what is frustration if not anger at being subjected to more displeasure than you think you've deserved? (The same kind of anger is what sends us inside for a beer when the lawn mower won't start. We're looking for compensation.)

- You've turned down an invitation to go someplace delicious for lunch because you're on a diet. So what happens that night? An "I earned it" second helping of mashed potatoes at dinner; an "I earned it" plate of cheese and crackers while watching T.V.; and maybe even a "what the heck, I'm going to be skipping lunch again tomorrow" ham-and-cheese on rye before bed. (You'd have been better off not to have skipped lunch in the first place. Compensation can be fattening.)
- You've had one of those days at work that has left you thoroughly drained. "And I'm supposed to torture myself with *exercise* after a day like this?" you say to yourself as you answer the call of your easy chair instead.

The human body, in a word, is an equation—one that is evolutionarily programmed to want to come out even. For every "minus" there must be a "plus" in order for us to keep from feeling cheated. So if and when you ever get totally plastered after being fired, console yourself that you are merely answering your body's primordial call for fair play.

1/
Your Bad Habit—How Bad Is It?

The medical profession means well, but it has a way of short selling our individuality. So its approach to keeping us well has been to discover that something is bad for some of us, predict that it is bad for most of us, and then proceed to issue warnings that scare the living daylights out of *all* of us.

At least one doctor, however, has been willing to stand up for our anatomical idiosyncrasies. "There can be little doubt that the statement 'all men are created equal' applies to voting rights and other dimensions of legal status, and to little else."

John L. Roglieri, M.D., was kind enough to say that, and what he's referring to is why the 130-pound Uncle Herbies of the world can indiscriminately indulge in coconut custard pie while others of us can't even butter our toast. No two vices affect any two people in precisely the same way. Which is why not all heavy drinkers get cirrhosis of the liver, and not all smokers get lung cancer. Smoking and drinking merely increase the *odds* of these things happening, just as obesity increases the *odds* of heart disease, and careless driving increases the *odds* of dying in a car accident.

This is not free license for us to let our hair down to our knees, however. The dangers of life's little pleasures are dose-related. The more we do, the more we risk.

Dr. Roglieri has written a book on that fact—called, appropriately, *Odds on Your Life* (Seaview, 1980)—and it's a statistical masterpiece. He consulted an exhaustive array of mortality statistics in putting together the accompanying tables. Read them and weep, or rejoice, whichever your particular level of indulgence may call for. Keep in mind, though, that these are statistical predictions, only. Your individual case may be helped—or hurt, for that matter—by your genetic inheritances. If many of your relatives are on record for having succumbed to vice-related disorders, you might want to view the risks of your own merrymaking accordingly.

4

Risks of Inactivity

Risk of Death from	Exercise Level			
	vigorous	moderate	some	none
Heart attack	1.0	1.3	1.9	2.3

NOTE: 1.0 represents the degree of risk for the exerciser.

Risks of Smoking

Risk of Death from	Smoking Level (cigarettes per day)			
	1-9	10-19	20-30	Over 40
Heart attack	1.0	1.4	1.8	2.2
Lung cancer	1.0	3.2	4.8	5.0
Bronchitis/ emphysema	1.0	1.3	1.7	2.1
Pneumonia	1.0	3.0	3.0	3.0
Stroke	1.0	1.5	1.5	1.5

NOTE: 1.0 represents the degree of risk for a nonsmoker.

Risks of Drinking

Risk of Death from	Drinking Level (drinks per week)					
	0	1-2	2-6	7-24	25+	alcoholic
Cirrhosis	1.0	2.0	10.0	20.0	50.0	125.0
Motor vehicle accident	1.0	1.0	2.0	4.0	10.0	10.0
Pneumonia	1.0	1.0	1.0	2.0	3.0	3.0

NOTE: 1.0 represents the degree of risk for a nondrinker.

Risks of Being Overweight

Risk of Death from	Weight Level			
	average weight	20 percent overweight	50 percent overweight	60 percent overweight
Heart attack	1.0	1.2	1.6	1.9
Diabetes	1.0	1.5	3.2	3.5
Hypertensive heart disease	1.0	1.1	1.5	1.9

NOTE: 1.0 represents the degree of risk for the nonobese.

SOURCE: Reprinted from *Odds on Your Life* by John Roglieri. Copyright 1980 by John Roglieri. Reprinted with permission of PEI Books, Inc. (All "Risk" tables in this chapter are derived from this same source.)

Risks of Stress Mismanagement

Risk of Death from	Mismanaged Stress from					
	drinking	depres-sion	high blood pressure	obesity	high blood fats	smoking
Heart attack	1.0	1.0	1.7	1.3	1.7	2.2
Motor vehicle accident	5.0	1.0	1.0	1.0	1.0	1.0
Cirrhosis	5.0	1.0	1.0	1.0	1.0	1.0
Suicide	1.0+	2.5	1.0	1.0	1.0	1.0
Lung cancer	1.0	1.0	1.0	1.0	1.0	2.0
Stroke	1.0	1.0	2.3	1.0	1.5	1.2

NOTE: 1.0 represents the degree of risk for one who copes effectively.

Risks of Driving

Driving Habits	Risk of Death from Motor Vehicle Accident
Drinking and Driving	
nondrinker	1.0
moderate drinker*	2.0
heavy drinker†	4.0
excessive drinker‡	10.0
Miles Driven per Year	
10,000	1.0
20,000	2.0
30,000	3.0
Use of Seat Belt	
always used	1.0
80 percent used	1.2
60 percent used	1.3
40 percent used	1.5
20 percent used	1.7
never used	1.8

NOTES: *Two to six drinks per week.
†Seven to twenty-four drinks per week.
‡Twenty-five plus drinks per week.
1.0 represents the degree of risk for the careful driver.

2/
How to Improve Your Chances of Cutting Down—on Anything

If Dr. Roglieri's statistics have had a sobering effect on you, you might (again?) be thinking about quitting or at least cutting down a particular indulgence. It's a decision only you can make, however, because only you know how much pleasure (and/or feelings of guilt) your bad habits give you. If your high times are beginning to conjure more foul thoughts than fair, though, you might think about making some changes. How good can cigarettes taste, after all, if with every puff your mental image of your lungs grows darker?

We've come up with some basic rules for helping you in the event you do decide to tone down, and we think they have a fair chance of working because they're well rooted in the pleasure principle outlined in chapter 1. Your body, remember, is a stickler for justice. You can't expect to get away with cheating it out of its evolutionarily ingrained quota for pleasure. Or at least not for very long. So . . .

Before you can quit or cut down on anything, you'd better have something else pleasurable to put in its place. That's rule number one for modifying potentially unhealthful behavior. Rule number two is:

Don't try to quit or cut down on anything until you've decided you really want to. We don't lack self-control when we raid the refrigerator; what we really lack is the honesty to admit that our double-decker sandwiches are still more important to us than our double-decker waistlines. We never really decided to control ourselves in the first place. Which brings us to rule number three:

Do not think that "willpower" is the answer. For a chosen few it might be, but for most of us, our bodies exert as much influence on us as our minds. And it's a good thing because in many cases our bodies have a better idea of what's right. The use of willpower, moreover, implies an element of conflict, one that would be better either to compromise or to resolve. If, for example, you think that to lose weight you have to give up the things you love, you would be smarter to cut back on things that are *not* so close to your heart. (I helped an ice cream-loving friend of mine lose weight once by suggesting he keep his ice cream but stop eating his chicken and fish fried—which we discovered was 7 giving him indigestion anyway.) Take the time to learn your priorities, in other words, and do your best to stick to them. But . .

Do not take relapses personally. It's not that you haven't meant well; it's just that you bit off more than you could chew. Take the time to map out a road to correction that isn't too hard to follow. Because by straying from your plan, you only lower your self-esteem. And self-esteem is perhaps your most important ingredient for success. Rule number five:

Avoid tempting situations, but only up to a point. We don't buy the theory that all social gatherings should be shunned to help you quit whatever it is you do at those affairs, because that sort of restraint only adds insult to injury. Do be careful, though. Peter Miller, Ph.D., author of *Personal Habit Control* (Simon and Schuster, 1978), reports that 25 percent of problem drinkers fall short of their goals due to "social pressure from friends." Smoking also tends to get encouraged at social events, so when you step out, do so with extra conviction. Rule number six:

Break a Bad Habit: Stop Being a Perfectionist

If you want to break a bad habit, or start a good one, about the worst thing you can be is a perfectionist. Because when you set your goals too high, you're likely to jump ship rather than fall short.

A better thing to be is an opportunist. Because as an opportunist, you gain confidence and pick up momentum from accomplishments that—to the perfectionist—might seem like failures. A few examples:

You want to give up smoking. As a perfectionist, you abandon the effort the first time you fail at going "cold turkey." As an opportunist, on the other hand, you view an occasional relapse against the amount you *used* to smoke and you feel buoyed by your progress.

You want to take up running. As a perfectionist, you get no further than the nearest fire hydrant before feeling "unacceptably inefficient." As an opportunist, you calculate how many calories your feeble first efforts earn you, and you reward yourself accordingly.

Dieting. As a perfectionist, you let one small slip become a landslide, somehow rationalizing a gorge as rightful punishment for a minor misdemeanor. As an opportunist, you stand tall after a slip, wisely recalling the day when that *one* potato chip used to be ten.

As you can see, trying to be perfect can keep you from being good.

Choose a time that is relatively stress-free. It can be physically and emotionally exhausting to quit something. So choose a time—a vacation, for example, or a lull in your schedule—that is going to allow you the energy and time for the other forms of pleasure you're going to need to counterbalance your "loss." Rule number seven:

Try to make your life more rewarding in other ways. Being wrapped up in bad habits is often a sign that we're not wrapped up in enough good ones. Indeed, boredom can cause us to reach for gusto in some dark places. Rule number eight:

Don't be afraid to try healthy substitutes. By that we mean reaching for something other than a triple Scotch after a crummy day at the office. Try reaching instead for a softball glove. Or an FM radio dial. Or the telephone, to make dinner reservations for two. Not all pleasures have to lead down paths of ruin. And finally . . .

Try giving rather than taking. Perhaps the "me" generation has run its course. Which may be why, even after all we've done to fulfill ourselves over the past decade, so many of us still feel empty. Possibly the answer to self-fulfillment doesn't lie in "self," after all, but rather in the satisfaction of knowing we've helped fulfill someone else.

3/
What's Not So Boring about Moderation

If the word *moderation* has a sour ring to it, it's because not enough people have given it a fair chance. We have a way of rushing right into abuse, thinking that if some feels good, more is going to feel better. Such, unfortunately, is not the case.

It's time moderation got the fair shake it deserves, because with a little bit of practice it can be a lot of fun. More fun than abuse, in fact, because instead of numbing the senses, moderation excites them. If you don't think so, think back on what got you interested in your current vice (or vices) in the first place.

Wasn't it the uniqueness of your first few experiences with it, and the new perspective it gave you on things? And it didn't take much, did it? Maybe just a couple of beers. Or one good hit on a Marlboro. Those were the good old days.

Now maybe you're into two manhattans before lunch, or a couple of smokes before breakfast—just to clear the cobwebs. Where did you go wrong?

You didn't really. Because at the heart of your escalating intakes have probably been good intentions. You've simply been trying to recapture those initially very positive and energizing feelings that relatively moderate intakes used to give you. But bad habits, you see, have a way of reaching points of diminishing return. By increasing your intake, you have actually been decreasing your chances of reliving those highs of old. Take alcohol, for example.

In very small doses, alcohol is a central nervous system stimulant. In slightly greater amounts it becomes a relaxant. But in large quantities it becomes a depressant. And that's bad because depressants can rob the body of energy, good spirits, and reason. Hardly the reasons you took to alcohol in the first place.

Nicotine also undergoes a dose-related metamorphosis. Initially a central nervous system stimulant, it can, in time, begin to numb the very abilities smokers claim that it excites. The ability to concentrate, for example. Studies at the University of Edinburgh in Scotland have shown that heavy smokers do less well than nonsmokers on memory tests. In the words of Columbia University psychologist Stanley Schachter, Ph.D., "The heavy smoker gets nothing out of smoking. He smokes only to prevent withdrawal" (*Annals of Internal Medicine,* January, 1978).

Coffee?

Same story. If you're drinking more than about three cups a day to steady your nerves, your coffee drinking could be what's responsible for those nerves in the first place. "High doses of caffeine . . . can produce . . . symptoms that are indistinguishable from those of anxiety neurosis," writes John F. Greden, M.D., in the *American Journal of Psychiatry* (October, 1974). With a bad habit, the secret is to catch and enjoy it at its peak.

How can you know where that peak occurs?

By paying attention. And by making a pact with yourself not to indulge in order to escape. Because in that case numbness is the goal—and addiction can be the result.

No, moderation need not be as great a comedown as you might think. By dispensing with the guilt that weighs on us when we overindulge, moderation can even be a new high—one that we can live with. As a 103-year-old skier is reported once to have told the *New York Times:*

"The secret to long life is to stay busy, get plenty of exercise, and don't drink too much. Then, again, don't drink too little."

Pleasure is an essential ingredient to health, but we defeat its purpose by overdosing to get it. As a corollary to Thoreau's remark about "that man" being "richest whose pleasures are the cheapest," we might add that "that man" is apt to be healthiest, too.

The Way We Were

There's a statement we should all be careful about making because the more we make it, the more it's apt to become true. It goes like this: "Well, that's just the way I am."

It comes in real handy when we're told we have a bad habit of putting things off. Or trying to do too many things at once. Or being forgetful. Or inconsiderate. Or late.

I found myself saying it the other day. I won't go into why, but soon after the words left my mouth, it suddenly occurred to me: *Why* is that just the way I am? I don't *like* being that way. It causes me stress. And I know nobody else is particularly happy about it.

It's amazing how willing we are sometimes to sell ourselves short. And out of sheer convenience, too.

So I decided to stop saying, "That's just the way I am." And I'm going to do my best to stop thinking it, too. Who knows, maybe I'll soon be able to say, "That's just the way I was."

4/

Alcohol: It Can Be a Tonic or a Poison

I once had the pleasure of conversing with a gentleman at the bar who told me that it was not unhealthful to drink because every living thing in the world can be turned into alcohol: ". . . flowers, grass, vegetables, bumblebees, *even you and me.*"

Those were his examples, not mine, and the point he went on to make (more fluently than I might have expected from a man in his condition) was that anything containing carbohydrates *could,* conceivably, be either fermented or distilled into ethanol.

When I good-naturedly questioned the palatability of sour mash bumblebees, he proceeded to lecture me that alcohol has been around for a very long time. So long, in fact, that it should be considered "an essential nutrient in the human diet."

At that point I got the feeling it was getting late. Which it wasn't, but I excused myself anyway.

I do that from time to time—go out for the express purpose of talking about health with "real" people. It keeps me on my toes, a little like wrestling somebody who doesn't know how to wrestle. You get a lot of elbows and knees.

Well, this guy's elbow was still sticking in my head the following day when I got to work, so I called an anthropologist from the University of Texas. And what Vaughn Bryant, Ph.D., told me was that yes, alcohol is likely to have been discovered some time ago (probably thirty-five hundred years before the birth of Christ) and that yes, in all likelihood it was consumed by our prehistoric ancestors, if not regularly, at least in occasional excess. During rituals and the like.

Notice, however, the word *occasional.* The cave person who woke up with a head full of rocks is not likely to have been much good at felling woolly mammoths or anything else, for that matter. The hangover was as much a warning signal then as it is now. It meant, quite simply, a compromise in one's efficiency and, hence, ability to survive.

Not that an occasional blowout is going to kill you. If it accomplishes—emotionally—what you had intended for it to accomplish, then not even your liver (an amazingly forgiving organ) is going to hold it against you. But . . .

Start to get squashed too often and you do invite trouble: liver disease, heart attack, cancer of the mouth, gout, obesity, pneumonia, diabetes, crashing your car, and losing your job, to name the most likely.

Alcohol can be a tonic—or it can be a poison.

Statistics published by the United States government in its *Second Report on Alcohol and Alcoholism* (U.S. Department of Health, Education, and Welfare, 1974) reveal that moderate drinkers are likely to outlive teetotalers. But they also show that abstainers are likely to last longer than those of us who drink to excess.

The magic word is moderation. That's six ounces (four jiggers) of 80-proof spirits a day if you're into the hard stuff, or 20 ounces of wine if grapes are your pleasure. Beer? Hold it to 4½ 12-ounce bottles.

Some researchers feel that nearly *twice* these amounts are safe, if consumed as part of a nutritionally adequate diet. But "such a generous limit should not be allowed for all people," says William J. Darby, M.D., Ph.D., a biochemist from Vanderbilt University and president of the Nutrition Foundation in New York. "Individual factors such as patterns of intake, general health, body weight and nutritional status can all determine the effect of alcohol on a person's system."

How can you know what's safe for you?

You can't for sure, but your feelings of general well-being should provide you with some indication.

"As medical investigators accumulate additional data on the effects of varying amounts of 'moderate' levels of consumption, more precise guidelines will be possible," Dr. Darby says. But until then, a limit of about six ounces of 80-proof liquor probably ought to be your daily maximum. As for those times when you go therapeutically overboard, well . . .

As stated, the liver is a very recuperative organ. You do impair its function somewhat by asking it to process too much alcohol too fast (for exactly how the liver deals with alcohol, see page 218), but it has the ability to bounce back in about a day for most people.

And what about the effects of *regular* daily drinking on the liver?

It's not as hard on it as binges are, as long as it's in moderation, according to Thurman Booker, D.O., head of medical development at Eagleville Hospital in Pennsylvania. A healthy liver can detoxify about one shot of 100-proof liquor an hour. It's when you go repeatedly flooding the thing that you increase its chances of going under. It takes the body about a week to totally clear itself of the toxic aftermath of an all-out drunk, so keep that in mind the next time you're tempted to give in to a little bit of the hair of the dog the morning after. Drinking for an occasional high is one thing; indulging just to break even is another.

"The sustained, immoderate drinking of spirits in any form can lead to a series of biochemical and physiologic deviations which can result in a variety of disorders of the CNS [central nervous system], liver, gastrointestinal tract, endocrine system [responsible for hormones], and skin," notes Sidney Cohen, M.D., in *Postgraduate Medicine* (December, 1978). "Chronic exposure to high doses of alcohol results in a state of physical dependence, with a resulting abstinence or withdrawal syndrome when ethanol ingestion is stopped abruptly." People have *died* from delirium tremens (DTs).

Now the good news: Yes, it's true alcohol can reduce your chances of dying of a heart attack. First, some statistics:

In a recent study by Arthur L. Klatsky, M.D., at the Kaiser-Permanente Medical Center in Oakland, California, it was found that among the 120,000 people evaluated, those who drank moderately were 30 percent less likely to have heart attacks than were teetotalers. Independent of age, sex, or prior related disease, even people good for six or more drinks a day had fewer heart attacks than abstainers (*Annals of Internal Medicine,* August, 1981).

In a six-year study of 7,705 Japanese men living in Hawaii, Katsuhiko Yano, M.D., found current drinkers to have the lowest incidence of heart attacks (30 cases per thousand), while former drinkers had the highest (56 per thousand). Teetotalers this time (at 44 heart attacks per thousand) fell about midway in between (*New England Journal of Medicine,* August 25, 1977).

Now, some facts:

Alcohol *appears* to encourage the development of high-density lipoproteins (HDLs)—a type of cholesterol—in the blood, which is good because HDLs seem to have the ability to keep *low*-density lipoproteins (LDLs)—the "bad" type of cholesterol—from accumulating on artery walls. Exercise has been shown to demonstrate the same ability, so if you really want to keep your heart happy, *earn* those two drinks a day.

Then there are the psychological benefits. "It's not the most potent therapeutic drug in the world," says Jonathan O. Cole, M.D., head of psychopharmacology at McLean Hospital in Massachusetts, "but I think alcohol has a mild anxiety-relieving, mood-elevating effect on a fair number of people."

A study done during the late sixties with senior citizens would seem to bear Dr. Cole out. Under the guidance of Robert Kastenbaum, Ph.D., director of the Adult Development and Aging Program at Arizona State University, beer was served six afternoons a week to geriatric patients at Cushing Hospital in Framingham, Massachusetts. Within two months, the percentage of people who could walk increased from 21 to 74 percent, group activity more than tripled, and there was a substantial reduction in the prescription of mood-altering drugs (*Alcohol and Old Age,* Grune and Stratton, 1980).

"It is encouraging to note that not everything one enjoys in life predisposes to cardiovascular disease," remarked William B. Kannel, M.D., in an editorial accompanying the Yano report in the *New England Journal of Medicine.* "There is nothing to suggest, for the present, that we must give up either coffee or alcohol in moderation to avoid a heart attack."

Moderation. The word keeps popping up. If moderation could *not* be said to describe your current patterns of alcohol intake, however, you might want to consider the following suggestions for cutting down. They come from the book *Drinking to Your Health* (Reston, 1981) by John A. Ewing, M.D., from the University of North Carolina.

- First off, he says, "When taking a drink, remember that you are taking a 'fix' of your favorite drug." Keep in mind the dangers of drinking too much, and chances are you won't.
- Try to determine in advance (when you're *sober*) how much you are going to drink, and do your best to stick to it.
- Use a jigger to accurately measure your drinks, and avoid the all-too-accommodating service of a heavy-handed host.
- Use mixers whenever possible, something noncarbonated with some food value, if you can.
- "Sip and savor your drinks." Remember, more than a couple is going to be bad for you. So enjoy what you can.
- Try to put a time limit on your drinking. Two hours should be tops.
- Think of getting drunk as "something to be guilty and worried about." It is.
- Don't just drink. Engage in conversation, watch television, or read while you sip.
- Never drink out of boredom. Think of alcohol as something to *enhance* life, and it will.
- "At a party, sip your first drink over 30 minutes and take about the same time for the second. If there has to be a third drink, stretch it out until you leave. Never take a fourth."
- Feel guilty if you take a drink because you feel you need one.
- Learn to eye an immunity to hangovers with suspicion. It's a sign that your system is becoming more comfortable with a toxic substance than it should be.
- Surprise yourself occasionally by doing something other than taking a drink. Exercise, take a shower, proposition your spouse. You'll be *living* the lift that alcohol only fakes.

We're not saying don't drink. But we are saying drink with respect for alcohol's potential dangers. It is the nature of *all* addicting substances that they have the power to make us feel "right" at the precise moment we ought probably to start feeling wrong. Keep that in mind and there's no reason you can't be sipping chablis at 90.

Tips for Taking the Calories Out of—and Putting Nutrients into—Your Drinking

So the medical community seems in agreement that consuming moderate amounts of alcohol is not damaging—and may even be conducive—to our health. Moderate daily drinking, particularly in people who exercise, appears to have positive effects on HDL cholesterol levels. And alcohol's sedative qualities, if treated with respect, appear to be of psychological value as well.

Before you go proposing a toast to that, though, consider two things: First, the amount of alcohol we're talking about is not a lot—somewhere in the neighborhood of two drinks a day. Second, if you're substantially overweight, and not well nourished, those two drinks may *not* be okay. Because if there's an ultimate junk food, alcohol, unfortunately, is it. No protein. No carbohydrates. No fats. No vitamins. No minerals.

Just calories. And lots of them. At seven calories per gram, alcohol serves up more calories than protein and carbohydrate (each of which is good for four calories per gram) and two less than pure fat, which saddles us with nine calories per gram.

For you lovers of zombies and Black Russians, though, that's only the beginning, because mixers also have calories (see adjoining table). And usually, like alcohol, very empty ones.

A Look at the Calories in Our Cocktails

	Portion* (ounces)	Calories	Carbo- hydrates (grams)	Alcohol (grams)
Distilled Liquors				
Brandy, California	1	73	(NA)	10.5
Brandy, cognac	1	73	(NA)	10.5
Cider, fermented	6	71	1.8	9.4
Gin, rum, vodka, rye, scotch:				
80 proof	1½	104	0	15.0
86 proof	1½	112	0	16.2
90 proof	1½	118	0	17.1
94 proof	1½	124	0	17.9
100 proof	1½	133	0	19.1
Liqueurs/cordials:				
Anisette	⅔	75	7.0	7.0
Apricot brandy	⅔	65	6.0	6.0
Benedictine	⅔	70	6.6	6.6
Creme de menthe	⅔	67	6.0	7.0
Curacao	⅔	55	6.0	6.0

	Portion* (ounces)	Calories	Carbo- hydrates (grams)	Alcohol (grams)
Wines				
Champagne, domestic	4	85	3.0	11.0
Dessert, 18.8 percent alcohol by volume	4	137	7.7	15.3
Madeira	4	105	1.0	15.0
Muscatel/port	4	158	14.0	15.0
Red, California	4	85	(NA)	10.0
Sauterne, California	4	85	4.0	10.5
Sherry, dry, domestic	4	85	4.8	9.0
Table, 12.2 percent alcohol by volume	4	85	4.2	9.9
Vermouth, dry, French	4	105	1.0	15.0
Vermouth, sweet, Italian	4	167	12.0	18.0
Malt Liquors, American				
Ale, mild	12	148	12.0	13.1
Beer, Budweiser	12	150	12.8	13.2
Beer, light	12	96	2.8	12.1
Beer, Michelob	12	160	14.9	14.2
Beer, Natural Light	12	100	5.5	11.6
Cocktails				
Daiquiri	3	125	5.2	15.1
Eggnog, Christmas	4	335	18.0	15.0
Gin rickey	8	150	1.3	21.0
Manhattan	3	165	7.9	19.2
Martini	3	140	0.3	18.5
Mint julep	10	212	2.7	29.2
Old-fashioned	4	180	3.5	24.0
Planters punch	4	175	7.9	21.5
Rum sour	4	165	(NA)	21.5
Tom Collins	10	180	9.0	21.5
Whiskey sour	3	138	7.7	(NA)
Mixers				
Bitter lemon	4	64	14.1	0
Club soda	4	0	0	0
Cola	4	43	12.0	0
Collins mixer	4	42	10.8	0
Ginger ale	4	45	11.3	0
Orange juice	4	28	6.0	0
Tomato juice	4	24	5.2	0
Tonic water	4	44	11.0	0

NOTES: *Standard serving. Glass sizes: cordial, ⅔ ounce; brandy, 1 ounce; jigger, 1½ ounces; sherry, 2 ounces; cocktail, 3 ounces; wine, 4 ounces; champagne, 5 ounces.
NA—information not available.

SOURCE: Adapted from *Food Values of Portions Commonly Used*, 13th ed., by Jean A. T. Pennington and Helen Nichols Church. Copyright 1980. Reprinted with permission of Harper and Row, Inc.

What we're getting around to is this: Some alcoholic beverages are "healthier" than others, and if you're out to keep your drinking as "good" for you as possible, you might want to educate your tastes accordingly.

Beer is your best bet. Per ounce it has fewer calories than wine and hard liquor, and it actually has some food value. A 12-ounce bottle, for example, contains about a gram of protein, 13.7 grams of carbohydrate, 13.5 percent of an adult male's Recommended Dietary Allowance (RDA) of phosphorus, 10.2 percent of his RDA of magnesium, and about 2 percent of the RDA for calcium. There is some niacin in beer (about 12 percent of the RDA per 12 ounces) and even some riboflavin—about 7 percent of the RDA. Compare those figures with the goose eggs turned in by hard liquor (whiskey, rum, vodka, and gin) and you begin to see why beer is the beverage of choice of most athletes.

Wine doesn't speak all that poorly for itself, either. One 3½-ounce glass of table wine, for example, serves up about 2.6 percent of the RDA of magne-

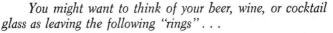

You might want to think of your beer, wine, or cocktail glass as leaving the following "rings" . . .

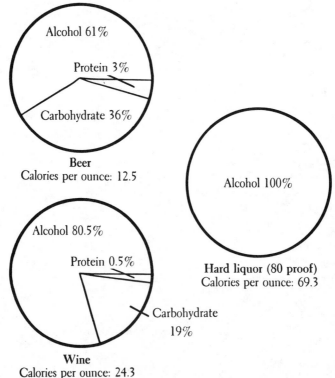

Beer
Calories per ounce: 12.5

Hard liquor (80 proof)
Calories per ounce: 69.3

Wine
Calories per ounce: 24.3

NOTE: The above percentages represent not volume or weight, but rather the percent of each beverage's *total calories* that come in the form of the nutrients listed.

sium, 1 percent of the RDA of calcium, 1.3 of phosphorus, and 4 percent of iron. Protein is admittedly scant (about a tenth of a gram per 3½-ounce glass) and carbohydrates are "so-so" at about 4.2 grams per 85-calorie serving.

As for the rest of the wide array of alcoholic beverages out there to serve you, we direct your attention again to our chart on drinks. It's sparse, we realize, but the science of nutrition just hasn't gotten around to analyzing the strawberry daiquiri.

Now some tips on getting a little more mileage—and a lot less calories—out of your hankering for hard liquor.

- Dilute with water or ice cubes as much as possible.
- Choose fruit juices as mixers rather than soft drinks.
- Beware of the double-jeopardy drinks (such as martinis and manhattans), which are booze on top of booze.
- Know that the sweetness in cordials usually comes from added sugar.
- So if it's dessert you want, there are fewer calories in a dish of ice cream than there are in a pina colada.

The Silicon Connection

Aside from vitamins, minerals, and calories, there may be yet another reason to choose wine and beer over hard liquor: a trace mineral called silicon.

An Austrian doctor reporting in the medical journal *Lancet* (May 17, 1980) cites evidence that deaths from heart disease are lowest in portions of England and Finland where silicon concentrations in drinking water are highest. Those statistics take on added significance, he says, in light of reports that atherosclerosis (hardening of the arteries) is more apt to occur in arteries that are silicon-deficient.

What's more, "the biological activity of silicon varies with its chemical form," the doctor reports, "and it would not be surprising if it were more active in a biological product such as wine than in its presumably inorganic form in drinking water.

"In wine-drinking countries, therefore, the dietary intake of silicon from wine may be one of the factors that contribute to favorable cardiovascular mortality. Beer contains similar concentrations of silicon, . . . which may help to explain why . . . beer consumption also seems to have a beneficial effect."

5/

Obesity: It's Not *What* You Weigh —It's Why

Is it really so unhealthful to be overweight?

That depends. Fat is like a police car in your rear view mirror—whether or not it's a cause for concern depends on why it's there. If you're carrying 20 extra pounds that owe themselves to alcohol abuse, a shoddy diet, and/or a lot of excuses not to exercise, then yes, they're hurting you. But if a slightly padded physique has stuck with you despite a prudent lifestyle, then don't worry about it. Results of a longevity study completed recently in Framingham, Massachusetts, suggest that there may be as many dangers associated with being too thin as too fat. As one M.D. felt obliged to comment on the findings: If left uncontested, they could "restore corpulence to its former esthetic glory."

Short of doing that, these latest statistics do at least make a point that our current obsession with thinness seems to have overlooked—namely, that *what* we weigh must be considered in light of *why* we weigh it. Anyone who smokes, to keep his weight down, for example, is robbing Peter to shortchange Paul.

Some of us are simply born with greater tendencies to put on weight than others, says George A. Bray, M.D., associate chief of the Division of Metabolism and Nutrition at Harbor/University of California at Los Angeles Medical Center. Dr. Bray has been doing research which seems to have put the finger on why some people can eat more than others. The reason is: brown fat. As opposed to white. All of us are born with some of each, says Dr. Bray, but those of us lucky enough to be born heavy on the brown side tend to be lean, because brown fat's job is to produce body heat by burning the calories that white fat stores.

"Brown fat makes up only about 1 percent of the body mass in most people," Dr. Bray told us. "But when it gets revved up, it can produce as much heat as the rest of the body can produce."

Brown fat, in other words, is a veritable blast furnace when it comes to obliterating calories. But it's impossible, unfortunately, to bolster the amount we're born with.

When we put on weight, we do so in the form of white fat, not brown, Dr. Bray says. What's worse, once a white fat cell has been created, it can't be destroyed. Shrunk, but not destroyed.

In light of this irreversibility, Dr. Bray emphasizes the importance of fighting obesity by never getting fat in the first place. A little pudgy is one thing, because white fat cells will grow in size before they will grow in number. But when we go bloating ourselves to the point where our existing cells can no longer handle the load, our bodies respond by making new ones. And a fat cell is a companion for life.

The brown fat theory makes sense. Not only does it explain why some people can eat more than others, it also explains why *all* of us tend to put on weight as we get older. Brown fat, researchers think, begins to lose its calorie-burning abilities as it ages. So the ice cream cones we could burn up as kids stick to our ribs when we become adults.

Some researchers see this metabolic slowdown as a protective device. George Mann, M.D., Ph.D., of the Vanderbilt University School of Medicine says: "There is no doubt that body fat is the best emergency ration we have." And so we tend to put more of it on as our chances of getting sick—and needing it—increase with age. "It's better to have 10 to 15 pounds of fat on your backside to live off when you're ill than to have to resort to total intravenous feeding," he says.

Fat, then, need not be the health hazard that slimming parlors would have us believe. As a ready supply of stored energy, it no doubt came to our rescue frequently along our bumpy evolutionary road.

But it mustn't be abused. Which it has been, unfortunately, and continues to be by an estimated 38 percent of adults in this country today.

Are you one?

You tell us. If your spouse has to cut your toenails and you dread getting in and out of your car, chances are the amount of extra weight you are carrying —for *whatever* reasons—is adversely affecting your health. It's hindering you physically, socially, and emotionally.

Obesity Hurts

One more reason not to be fat: It hurts. Not just socially, but physically. When neurophysiologists from France compared the pain thresholds of normal-weight women to those of a group 30 percent or more overweight, they found that the obese women were sissies by comparison. In proportion to their degree of obesity, they showed significantly "heightened sensitivities to pain," causing the researchers to speculate that obesity may reduce normal amounts of painkilling chemicals (enkephalins and endorphins) in the brain. These are the same chemicals, incidentally, that vigorous exercise promotes—hence the "runner's high," and marathoners who can truck on despite blistered feet.

A doctor will tell you you're too fat if you weigh "20 percent more than you should." But what's that?

A good question. Bone size and muscularity vary so much from person to person that an "ideal weight" for anybody is a clumsy estimate, at best. With that in mind, consider the following formulas:

For women:
Ideal body weight = 100 pounds + 4 pounds per inch above five feet.

For men:
Ideal body weight = 100 pounds + 5 pounds per inch above five feet.

What these equations fail to take into account is the all-important factor of lifestyle. A healthful one earns you the right to carry around more weight than an unhealthful one.

Why?

Let's look, first of all, at being physically active. If you're physically active, more of your excess poundage is apt to be in the form of muscle than fat. And muscle is less of a burden on the heart because it participates in its own transport. Fat, by comparison, takes a free ride. Then, too, by being physically active you prepare your heart for the extra demands that being pleasantly plump puts upon it. By allowing yourself to get heavy *without* being active, you create an unfair match between the capability of your heart and the amount of cargo you ask it to carry around.

Now smoking.

You can get away with carrying more fat around by not smoking because you allow your blood to transport oxygen as it should. When you smoke, you put carbon monoxide in your blood instead of oxygen, and it's oxygen, not carbon monoxide, that your heart needs to get you up a flight of stairs at 5'8", 240 pounds. Smoking also interferes with the blood in a way that makes blood fats more apt to stick to artery walls; and if you're overweight, chances are you have an overabundance of these fats for smoking to work its ill effects on. People who are overweight *in addition* to being smokers increase their chances of heart disease over people who are merely one or the other. Cigarettes and fat are a very unhealthful combination.

Being overweight, though, does not have to mean being unhealthy. However, there are certain limits to that decree, because by going overboard *too* much you put unnatural burdens on your body regardless of how healthfully you live. The heart, lungs, kidneys, pancreas, gallbladder, joints, feet—even the skin and reproductive organs—begin to buckle under too much weight.

And how much is that?

Studies indicate that anything over about 30 percent of ideal weight is where people begin to ask for trouble. People who are that much overweight are more apt to get diabetes, they are more accident prone, they run greater than normal risks from surgery and anesthesia, they are more susceptible to breast and prostate cancer, and they experience more emotional disorders. The human body simply was not designed to carry more than a certain quota of spare rations.

So view your physique with that in mind. Forget about fashion; think about health. Perhaps the best way to determine your ideal weight (providing you suffer from no serious glandular disorder) is simply to eat sensibly and exercise moderately for a year. If you don't like what you see after that, take solace in the fact that anatomical upholstery in ancient Rome was considered very chic. And that Peter Paul Rubens, rather than paint Cheryl Tiegs, would have preferred to render Miss Piggy.

6/

Food Cravings: Make Peace, Not War, with Them

Life is too short, and food too great a pleasure, to be forever cursing our appetites. And yet we do it all the time. The following confessions come from people quoted in the December, 1980, issue of the *Runner.*

> I'm always thinking about food. I can't think of a day when food hasn't somehow been a controlling factor. What to eat, where to eat, when to eat ... have I eaten too much? No other subject is so all-consuming, not even sex.
> —*A musician in his thirties who runs 30 to 40 miles a week to keep his weight down.*

> Basically I see myself as a glutton under control. I make choices because how I look is more important. If I gave up being conscious of my appetite, I would be fat.
> —*A filmmaker, age 34, who swims or runs two or more hours a day to keep on top of her physique.*

> The coffee wagon comes around at the office. I have a muffin. Then I go back 15 minutes later and have a jelly doughnut, then I want a chocolate bar. The effect is narcotic.
> —*A lawyer who is humbled by his craving for sweets.*

Once an ally and a pleasure, food has become an enemy and a source of stress for millions of us—a far cry, certainly, from the days when a full stomach was a goal as justifiable as survival itself. Our problems with food now range from anorexia nervosa (a form of self-starvation) to morbid obesity. So uneasy have we become about food, in fact, that the manager of a posh New York City restaurant recently complained that his restrooms were becoming postfeast vomitoriums for the fashionably thin. Where did we go wrong?

We didn't, really. Our environment did. Progress put us behind desks instead of mules. And modern technology made our food more fattening (through refinement) at the same time it made it more available. The result has been the ten or so extra pounds that now have us resenting rather than relishing

our dinners.

What can we do about it?

Try to re-create the days of old. "We've got to get off diets as such and learn to live more normally with food," says Yale University psychologist Judith Rodin, Ph.D.

That means eating more of *what* we used to, the *way* we used to: wholesome foods, guilt-free.

"The classical and memorable meals out of our primitive past were the two- and three-day massive 'pig-outs' following the successful capture of a wild boar, antelope, or zebra," attest Bernhoff A. Dahl, M.D., and David Fingard,

Deny It Now, Gorge Later

Your appetite is like a bar of wet soap: The harder you try to control it, the more it's apt to get out of hand. That was demonstrated rather convincingly in a study by a psychologist at the University of London.

After examining the eating habits of 68 normal medical students, Jane Wardle found a connection between the degree to which students exercised "dietary restraint" and the degree to which they gave in to binges. She found, too, that the students who fought their appetites most were the most overweight.

The women in Ms. Wardle's group were more given to dietary restraints—and hence "binging"—than the men. They reported an average of 4.7 gluttonous episodes a month, compared to the men's 2.2. Binging was defined as "eating lots of food even when perhaps not hungry."

"Subjects of all weight classifications, if they were restricting their food intake, reported more eating binges, more craving, and more problems with stopping eating," Ms. Wardle said.

The message was clear: Deny it now, gorge later. But an interesting sidelight to come out of the study was that binging—even for the most "normal" eaters examined by Ms. Wardle—was surprisingly common: "as often as once a week," Ms. Wardle said. What seemed to separate the chronic (and hence, overweight) bingers from the normal ones, though, was how they *reacted* to their binges. The unrestrained eaters went on occasional splurges without much afterthought—but the dieters panicked, put even greater restrictions on themselves as a result, and only brought their next binge that much closer in the process.

The human appetite, in other words, does not take kindly to being thwarted. And why should it? After all, for thousands of years hunger was something we dedicated our lives to prevent.

M.D. These doctors have designed a diet plan around gorging (which they appropriately call the Pig-Out Diet). And perhaps its most salient contribution to the weight-losing community, Dr. Dahl told us, has been the message that eating one large meal a day doesn't *have* to be bad for you. In fact, our bodies and our minds are set up to do it quite nicely.

But we're also set up to nibble.

"In our prehuman past, several patterns of eating behavior succeeded each other," explain A. David Jonas, M.D., and Doris F. Jonas in *Modern Medicine* (May 15, 1976). As tree dwellers, we snacked on fruits. When we dropped to the ground, we took to nibbling on grasses and small amounts of scavenged meat. When we got our land legs together, we began ganging up on our own meat. And when we got our heads together, we mastered the arts of farming and animal husbandry that have allowed us to be the well-rounded gluttons we are today.

Vestiges of *all* of these phases, however, remain imprinted on our brains. Which is why we feel like nibbling sometimes—and gorging other times. "Human beings are heirs not only to genetic influences of the immediate past . . . but also to the whole developmental history of the species," the Jonases say. Keep that in mind the next time you get the munchies, or the uncontrollable urge for prime rib.

The human appetite, in short, is a complex force with a long and windy road behind it. And the closer scientists have tried to look at this force, the less they feel that any hard and fast rules can be made about how to control it. "Its multiple facets—both psychological and physiological—form such a complex phenomenon that the task of understanding seems nearly hopeless," wrote Gail McBride several years ago in the *Journal of the American Medical Association* (September 27, 1976). Ms. McBride was commenting on the findings of the Dahlem Conference of Appetite and Food Intake, an internationally attended symposium held in West Germany. Conference chairman Dr. J. Trevor Silverstone of London summed it up this way: "We all came clean for a change and admitted we still know very little."

In a way, that's saying a lot. Because what this bewilderment from the scientific community suggests is that no one's in a better position to deal with your appetite than you are. The Jonases have been believers in a hands-off approach all along.

"The tendency to regard overweight or underweight as a uniform manifestation . . . ignores the diversity of the many phylogenetic [evolution-caused] eating patterns that underlie the regulation of weight in the human species. It is hardly surprising that in these circumstances the physician's intervention so seldom achieves ideal results."

So what do they suggest?

"It is a recognized therapeutic principle that when you can't change a condition, you accept it and try to use it for the purpose at hand. The patterns involved in the condition of obesity ideally lend themselves to treatment on this basis."

What they're saying is that if you find it easier—more enjoyable—to contend with food just once a day, fine. And if you find that nibbling is more your style, that's okay, too. The important thing is to feel good about the way you eat. And knowing that there is no *right* or *wrong* way is the first step in doing that. "Three squares" a day is a relatively recent and arbitrary convention.

"Vast fortunes have been made writing and preaching about diet schemes and social clubs for weight control, as well as by selling gadgets, postal scales for weighing out minuscule portions, drugs, and memberships. None of these approaches, however, deals with man's basic nature—the urge to consume food abundantly whenever available," write Drs. Dahl and Fingard in their book, *The Pig-Out Diet.*

But won't that just keep you fat? you must be wondering. Not if you eat the right foods. Aha—a catch after all! you say.

Not really. Because eating healthful foods should not feel oppressive when made part of an "eat-all-you-want, when-you-want" program. The caveman, remember, did not pig out on chocolate mousse. Nor did he forage for potato chips.

If large, infrequent meals are going to be your style, stick to lean meats, vegetables, low-fat dairy products, complex carbohydrates (potatoes, brown rice, beans), and fresh fruit. If you're going to nibble your way healthy, go for fresh vegetables (carrots, celery, cauliflower, broccoli, and the like), cheese, and anything else you can manage out of the gorger's list just noted.

Sweets?

Sure. But in moderation. Make yourself happy enough on healthy stuff, though, and you might—like the caveman—not miss them at all.

Make peace, not war, with your appetite. Experiments with rats and humans at Emory University in Atlanta, Georgia, have shown that when pain is inflicted, many rats—and many people—will overeat or indulge in some other bad habit. Psychologist Michael Cantor, Ph.D., has observed that a pinch to a rat's tail, for example, will cause it to eat more grain, even after its had its fill.

So stop pinching yours. Find a healthful meal plan that feels good—the way food was meant to.

7/

How to Make It Healthier
to Go Out to Dinner

Ninety percent of the people who lose weight wind up gaining most of it back because they go on diets that fail to consider the simple evolutionary fact that the human body was not designed to feel deprived.

It was designed to feel good. Feeling good is what the survival instinct is all about. It's why you goofed on the grapefruit diet. And it's why you'll goof again—on any diet that denies your body its inalienable right to feel satisfied.

"Gosh, we'd love to join you for dinner, but . . . well, I'm on a diet."

Sound familiar? Those are very dangerous words, because he who speaks them will very likely stay at home and consume many low-sodium pretzels before giving in to a 1,200-calorie "just a sandwich" (made with diet bread and imitation mayonnaise) before calling it a night. Psychologists call it compensation. We call it stuffing the sorrows.

If going out to dinner used to be a pleasurable and relaxing experience for you—which you now miss because you're on a diet—go to the phone right now and make reservations at your favorite restaurant. There is no reason that you can't (by adhering to the following game plan) come home feeling relaxed, rewarded, guilt-free, and (best of all) satisfied.

The important thing to remember is that buried beneath every menu's fattening language is some basic food, food that you and your diet have been very comfortable with at home. There are dishes in cream sauces that may approach a thousand calories, but there are also seafood items that needn't sting you for more than about two hundred. It's up to *you* to be able to tell them apart.

Ready to order?

For your appetizer, steer clear of items that are either sauteed or heavily sauced. A good choice here is the shrimp cocktail.

If you order a salad, make sure to ask if it comes already dressed. If so, request it be stripped down. Order either half the amount of dressing normally served, or be really brave and specify a concoction of your own: lemon juice and

28

vinegar, or tomato juice and vinegar, or all three. Experiment at home with proportions so that you sound committed when you order. And stand firm if your waiter rolls his eyes. A good restaurant should offer good service, right?

For your entree, don't be fooled by something that starts with a reasonably innocent base such as fish, chicken, or veal. These relatively low-calorie meats are the ones most apt to arrive bullied by some high-calorie casserole or sauce. Be bullish yourself; ask what the chef has in mind for your main dish before you order it.

Many times you're best off with a cut of beef that doesn't need any high-calorie help—either a lean cut of steak (broiled), or ground sirloin. In descending order, red meat looks like this on the calorie chart: prime rib is the most fattening, followed by T-bone steak, porterhouse steak, club steak, sirloin steak, ground sirloin, round steak, and flank steak. Avoid eating any visible fat, and steer clear of jumbo portions.

Fish is usually your best bet—broiled, *not fried.* (Anything that survives deep frying picks up needless fat in addition to calories, particularly if it's been breaded.) Cod, haddock, and flounder are less fattening than bass, halibut, and salmon. Lobster is a good choice—without the butter, of course. Butter contains 36 calories per pat which, melted, translates to about four hundred calories for a little quarter-cup (two-ounce) container—more calories than the lobster has.

The entrees, then, to look for are: lean cuts of beef, fish (easy on the butter), baked chicken (not fried), liver (if you don't mind swabbing it of excess grease), and shellfish (broiled rather than breaded).

Compared to your entree, vegetables are easy. Anything green is fair game. Baked potatoes are also legal. Avoid anything "creamed" and beware (as with your appetizer) of anything "sauteed."

Dessert? No problem if they're serving melon or some other fresh fruit. Otherwise, you're out of luck.

What can you save by all this? About one thousand calories. Skip the before-dinner cocktail and disappoint the wine steward, and you can do even better than that.

If our approach to eating out sounds a bit stark, then decorate it a bit. Chances are, though, that in the plush atmosphere of a good restaurant you won't have to. It's those lonely nights spent moping over T.V. reruns and low-sodium pretzels that can lead to gluttony.

The Better the Restaurant, the Better Your Chances

Nothing against diners that welcome truckers, but when it comes to having some control over what you order, you usually get what you pay for. Not that Joe on the grill doesn't *want* to be more accommodating. He can't. Many of his entrees come to him ready-made, wanting little more from Joe than some heat and a sprig of parsley.

If you're going to be pushy, go to a place that can give. Food "made to order" means just that, which is why it takes so long. Play your cards right, though, and you can make that wait worth your while.

Things like Lobster Newburg—hold the Newburg. You'll be amazed at what you can get away with. The secret is to be *very* polite, almost apologetic. Preface your order with remarks like, "I know you're going to think I'm crazy, but . . ."

Head for the Salad Bar but Not the Chef's Salad

Don't be fooled by the bouquet of lettuce; a chef's salad is a meal. And a big one. Topped with turkey, roast beef, ham, cheese, a hard-boiled egg, and a few olives, what most dieters order as an exercise in restraint is more like an act of indulgence.

The average chef's salad tips the scales at about a thousand calories—and that's in the nude. Dress one of the feasts in a five-tablespoon suit of something Russian, blue cheese, or Italian, and you're looking at 1,400—a figure that dwarfs a lot of full-course meals.

If it's a salad you want, keep the chef out of it. Many restaurants nowadays offer salad bars, and they're a dieter's dream come true. "Rights" to one rarely costs more than four dollars, and for all they offer in the way of wholesome, low-calorie food, they can be a real bargain.

Pack away all the greens you want. For sources of protein, look to cottage cheese, garbanzos (chick-peas), kidney beans, and slices of hard-boiled egg. Some really good bars offer bean sprouts, green peppers, chopped mushrooms, cauliflower, and broccoli. Steer clear of the sweetly "pickled" stuff, and avoid concoctions that appear oily or laced with mayonnaise.

For a dressing, either go lightly with French (66 calories per tablespoon compared to 74 for Russian, 76 for blue cheese, 80 for Thousand Island, and 83 for Italian) or really play it thin and use just vinegar.

If the croutons appear unbuttered, toss in a handful of those. Parmesan cheese? A tablespoon at 23 calories can't hurt. Bacon bits? Go easy, even on the fake ones.

Depending on your choice of components, the salad you make for yourself shouldn't cost you more than about six hundred calories—probably *less than half* of what the chef's salad gets. And if you're not quite satisfied after your first creation, wander back for more. It's better to top off your appetite with celery than with bread sticks.

The Vocabulary of Haute Cuisine

For those of you who enjoy French restaurants, we offer the following mini-lesson to help you make sense of what you're liable to run into:

Ail is garlic; *au gratin* means with cheese and bread crumbs; *beurre* is

(*continued on page 34*)

Yes, Fast Food Is Fattening

Dining out with the Kings and the Colonels of the fast-food industry can have its advantages. Good nutrition, however, is rarely one of them.

Where do the foods at these restaurants go wrong? That depends on the food. Some—like the "milk" shakes that consist largely of vegetable fats—go wrong right from the start. Others—like the hamburgers that start out using beef leaner than ground chuck—get dealt a foul blow later, when it comes time for "fixin's." Basically, some of the food is reasonably healthful. But "basically" is seldom how it enters our mouths.

The biggest food-offender at your local hamburger hop is the deep fryer. And in the worst way—with saturated (possibly rancid) hydrogenated vegetable oil. Or worse yet, lard. A piece of fish, worth all of a hundred calories before going in, can emerge from a bath of hot oil toting twice that many.

Then there are the beverages and the desserts—big money makers for the restaurant, but big losers for you. Most eight-ounce soft drinks are good for about one hundred calories, all of them virtually nutrient-free. And what many of these places are calling "milk" shakes are in fact ingenious imitations, collections of nondairy ingredients that offer few of the nutrients, yet *twice the calories* of milk.

We will admit, though, that a Big Mac, or a Quarter Pounder, or a Whopper is *not* junk food. It is, however, a whopping lot of calories. And fat. Some fast-food entrees, for that matter, can be nearly *50 percent fat.* Chalk that up against the 30 percent levels now being recommended by the federal government and you can see that the "break" you deserve —"today" or any day—deserves restraint.

Percentage of Calories from Protein, Carbohydrate, and Fat

Most nutritionists agree that an ideal diet would derive about 15 percent of its calories from protein, 55 percent from carbohydrate, and not more than about 30 percent from fat (as little saturated as possible).

Note how the different cuisines compare to this ideal. If the percentages don't add up exactly to 100, it's because we did some rounding off in arriving at them. But the message is clear, nonetheless: French and American meals tend to be lopsided in fat, while Italian, Chinese, Mexican, and Middle Eastern fare come considerably closer to what nutritionists recommend.

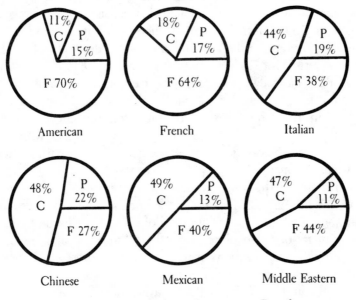

NOTE: C = carbohydrate, P = protein, F = fat.

Nutritive Content of Select Ethnic Menus

	American	French	Italian	Chinese	Mexican	Middle Eastern
Calories	1,770	1,341	941	1,247	512	1,404
Protein (grams)	67	57	44	70	16	37
Carbohydrates (grams)	48	62	103	151	63	165
Fat, saturated (grams)	70	49	13	16	9	32
Fat, unsaturated (grams)	68	47	27	22	14	36
Total fat (grams)	138	96	40	38	23	68
Cholesterol (milligrams)	338	430	162	257	35	242
Sodium (milligrams)	932	1,066	2,530	3,712	928	3,773
Potassium (milligrams)	1,944	2,063	1,599	1,410	861	1,479
Vitamin A (percent of RDA)	108	111	75	94	57	256
Vitamin C (percent of RDA)	152	154	88	71	87	252
Thiamine (percent of RDA)	30	44	45	112	24	90
Riboflavin (percent of RDA)	43	73	44	63	16	63
Niacin (percent of RDA)	78	96	49	87	26	55
Calcium (percent of RDA)	16	17	30	21	19	42
Iron (percent of RDA)	56	43	54	74	31	72
Phosphorus (percent of RDA)	70	66	55	77	25	56

NOTE: RDA—Recommended Dietary Allowances.

SOURCE: Pillsbury-Honeywell Nutrition Analysis System, 1981.

butter; *boeuf* is beef; *bouilli* means boiled; *canard* is duck; *caneton* is duckling; *champignons* are mushrooms; *creme* is cream; *farci* means stuffed; *frit* means fried; *gigot* is lamb; *gratine* means baked with bread crumbs; *grille* means broiled; *jambon* is ham; *legumes* are vegetables; a *mousse* can be almost anything thickened with cream; *nouilles* are noodles; *oeufs* are eggs; *pane* means breaded; *poche* means poached, *pommes de terre* are potatoes, *porc* is pork; *poulet* is chicken; a *quiche* can be almost anything in a pie crust; *riz* is rice; *salade* is salad; *saute* means fried in butter; a *souffle* is something that's had egg whites whipped into it; *veau* is veal; and *vin,* of course, is wine.

So what would *pommes de terre frites* be? Fried potatoes. Very good. Now that you can read the menu, you've got a fighting chance.

Yes, There Are Ethnic Differences

You can go American, French, Italian, Chinese, Mexican, or Middle Eastern. Which is apt to be the wisest decision nutritionally?

That's a question we asked a specially programmed computer. What we did was feed the computer representative recipes from each type of restaurant, and the numbers you see in the preceding box are what it came up with. These recipes won't parallel precisely the dishes you'll be confronting when you go out, but they should come fairly close. Ethnic cuisines have certain pet ingredients, and these are the ones we did our best to include in our selections. What we tested:

- **American:** a 12-ounce sirloin steak (broiled), a baked potato with sour cream, buttered broccoli, and a salad with Russian dressing.
- **French:** chicken and cream sauce, crusty molded potatoes, peas braised with onions, and a salad with French dressing.
- **Italian:** spaghetti with meat sauce, Italian bread, and a salad with Italian dressing.
- **Chinese:** chicken chow mein, wonton soup, a shrimp egg roll, and white rice.
- **Mexican:** two tacos, a cup of gazpacho soup, and a serving of fried rice.
- **Middle Eastern:** spinach-cheese pie, *hummus bi tahina* (chick-peas), Arab bread, rice, and a salad with oil dressing.

So put on your bifocals and start reading. We warn you now, though, that if it's fat you're trying to cut down on, quaint little French restaurants and juicy American steak houses offer jumbo portions of it. And if sodium is your fear, think twice about going Middle Eastern or Chinese.

As for the *good* things in the various ethnic cuisines we tested, trust that there are plenty of those, too. Going out to dinner *can* have its nutritional advantages.

8/

Tips for Sidetracking a Sweet Tooth

The next time you finish dinner but your mouth says, "I'm not done yet," try something: Instead of having some high-calorie dessert, have a piece of fresh fruit. And before you go wrinkling your nose, see if it doesn't:

- feel to your jaw muscles a little like a second helping of steak,
- feel to your sweet tooth a little like a piece of cake,
- and feel to your conscience like you've just saved a bushel of calories—which you have.

Fruit, like flattery and sex, is one of the few things in life that, in addition to being pleasurable, is good for us. It's time we restored it to its former irresistible glory.

"We evolved as fruit eaters," University of Texas anthropologist Vaughn Bryant, Ph.D., told us. "In certain climates, and at certain times of the year, I'd estimate that fruit made up as much as 50 percent of our prehistoric diet." Now we're lucky if we eat the piece we get stuck with in a packed lunch.

Why has fruit lost its punch?

Because sugar came along and spoiled our taste buds rotten. Dr. Bryant told us a story of children living on an isolated tropical island being offered modern-day candy; most of them simply didn't like it. Too sweet. We Americans would do well to react the same way.

On the contrary, though, the constant barrage of sugar that we get in our diets has upped our average annual intake 22 percent since 1900. Our consumption of fresh fruits since 1929, reflecting this changeover, has dropped 43 percent.

What has that meant for our bodies? Trouble. Obesity, diabetes, tooth decay, and heart disease have been on the rise during these sweet but sour years. "It may be surmised that abandonment of wild fruits as a dietary component may be responsible for some of the present-day health problems of modern man," reports John R. K. Robson, M.D., professor of nutrition and medicine at the Medical University of South Carolina (*Journal of Human Nutrition,* February, 1978).

We should be eating more fruit and less frosting, in other words. And here's why:

Fruit satisfies our sweet tooth *naturally*. It gives us sugar, but in a way and *at a pace* that our bodies have been designed to handle. (Refined sugar comes at us in too concentrated a form, the result of which can be feelings of weakness and actual hunger after the pancreas panics and produces more sugar-taming insulin than it should.) Fruit, because it has to be chewed and digested, and because it supplies its own natural sugar buffers in the form of fiber, provides the kind of gradual and *usable* energy boost that the twentieth century candy bar cannot. (You can prove that to yourself simply by having a large piece of fruit the next time you might ordinarily have candy or a piece of pastry to ward off between-meal hunger. You'll find you'll get a lot more mileage from the fruit.)

Metabolically speaking, then, our bodies spent millions of years getting energy from cantaloupes rather than candy bars—one of the reasons we were less obese in those days, too. A small piece of chocolate cake, which in a pinch you could put away in about a minute, provides close to three hundred calories. How long would it take you to eat four medium-size apples? Or eight small peaches? Or a quart and a half of strawberries? Same number of calories.

And what you get for those calories in fruit is this: ample amounts of vitamin C, a lot of important minerals, valuable supplies of fiber, and—for those of you worried about cholesterol—an effective cholesterol-lowering agent called pectin. (About all you get with the cake is a guilty conscience and chocolate lips.)

Pectin has been proven effective in lowering cholesterol counts in humans by an average of 13 percent. The amount required to do this is 15 grams daily. Oranges, bananas, cherries, grapes, tomatoes, peaches, and raspberries are good sources.

Then there are bioflavonoids, a group of substances prevalent in the pulp and rinds of fruit, which scientists have found do two things: strengthen capillary walls and make vitamin C more absorbable. Bioflavonoids are most abundant in citrus fruits but also travel in the company of apples, cherries, elderberries, currants, and the skins and leaves of most vegetables. Research has found that they can help prevent capillary bleeding, gynecological problems, diabetic cataracts, the common cold, and even arthritis. And, because their function is to help maintain the integrity of the capillary system (the network of tiny blood vessels responsible for transporting nutrients to individual cells), the therapeutic effects of bioflavonoids are far-reaching.

Last, but not least, your teeth. Fruit does contain some cavity-producing sucrose, but very little. It gets most of its sweetness from other kinds of sugar (fructose and xylitol) that cannot be used as easily by bacteria, and hence promotes cavities less than the likes of candy. Then, too, fresh fruit does its own brushing. Certain sticky versions—like dried apricots, figs, and raisins—can cause problems, but fresh fruit presents negligible cause for dental alarm. (Most varieties are only about 2 percent sucrose, whereas hard candy can go as high as 96 percent. Milk chocolate logs in at about 58 percent, and presweetened breakfast cereals are better than 50 percent sucrose.)

Considering that we cook most of the vegetables we eat, and bleach the flour in most of our breads, and unnaturally fatten most of our sources of meat protein, and add a host of preservatives to the majority of our dairy products, fruit stands out as the least adulterated of our basic food groups. Dr. Bryant

Fruits: Sweets That Make Sense

	Portion	Calories	Carbohydrates (grams)
Fruit			
Apple	1 medium	80	20
Apricots, fresh	3	55	14
Avocado	½	188	7
Banana	1 medium	101	26
Cantaloupe	¼ medium	41	10
Cherries, sweet	10	47	12
Grapefruit	½	40	10
Grapes	10	34	9
Honeydew melon	⅛	62	14
Orange	1 medium	64	16
Peach, peeled	1 medium	38	10
Pear	1 medium	100	25
Pineapple	½ cup	40	11
Plum	3 medium	63	17
Raisins	¼ cup	105	28
Strawberries	½ cup	28	6
Watermelon	1 slice	111	27
Other Sweets			
Boston cream pie	1 piece	208	34
Doughnut, cake-type	1 plain	227	30
Ice cream	1 cup	257	28
Milk chocolate bar	1 ounce	147	16

NOTES: *Per 100 grams of food cited.
RDA—Recommended Dietary Allowances.
NA—information not available.

paid fruit the compliment of being, "pound for pound, . . . one of the best ways to spend our calories."

So stop relegating fruit to centerpieces and brown paper bags. Eat it— often. And if you find yourself missing those demonic delights at first, just remember that a chocolate mousse would have turned a cave person green— with indigestion, not envy.

"In the beginning," dessert was good for us.

Dietary Fiber* (grams)	Vitamin A (percent of RDA)	Vitamin C (percent of RDA)	Potassium (milligrams)
5.7	2	10	152
1.9	58	18	301
2.0	7	27	680
3.4	5	20	440
1.0	92	75	341
1.5	1	12	129
0.6	2	62	132
0.9	1	3	87
0.9	2	72	470
2.0	5	110	263
1.4	27	12	202
2.3	1	12	213
1.2	1	22	113
2.1	5	5	144
6.8	trace	trace	277
2.2	1	73	122
(NA)	50	50	426
(NA)	3	trace	61
(NA)	1	trace	52
(NA)	12	2	241
(NA)	2	trace	109

SOURCES: Adapted from U.S. Department of Agriculture Handbook no. 456, and *McCance and Widdowson's The Composition of Foods*, by A. A. Paul and D. A. T. Southgate (New York: Elsevier/North-Holland Biomedical Press, 1978).

9/

The Pros and Cons of Coffee

Whether or not coffee is bad for you is a question that no one can answer better than you can. If you drink less than about three cups a day because you enjoy its flavor and respect its effects, then coffee is probably not doing you any harm. If, on the other hand, you drink considerably more than that because you feel you *have* to, just to get by, then coffee *is* bad for you and you ought to cut down. Here's why.

Consumed moderately, coffee can have a positive and very productive effect. Laboratory experiments have shown that judicious amounts of caffeine can speed reaction time and increase mental alertness, which is probably why we drink more coffee in this country than any other beverage. In addition to tasting good, it works.

But coffee has a darker side. As with alcohol, amount is all-important. In quantities greater than 250 milligrams (the amount in three to four cups of instant coffee), caffeine can cause headaches, irritability, sleeplessness, fatigue, and confusion—hardly the reasons we turn to it in the first place. In fact, too much coffee can drive you (slightly) crazy. "High doses of caffeine can produce pharmacological actions essentially indistinguishable from those of anxiety neurosis," concurs John F. Greden, M.D., in the *American Journal of Psychiatry* (October, 1974). Coffee, in other words, can turn Dr. Jekyl into Mr. Hyde.

Several years ago, the *American Journal of Psychiatry* (July, 1978) reported the case of a 28-year-old Alaskan trapper who—in an effort to remain "alert" during a 1,000-mile dog sled race—downed two cups of coffee, three cola drinks, and four Vivarin tablets within three hours. He proceeded to spend the next six hours in never-never land. Hallucinations, dizziness, and severe tremors caused him twice to topple from his sled.

An extreme example?

The trapper had taken in 1,000 milligrams of caffeine—not that far out of the ordinary, considering that two cups of coffee at breakfast, one for a 10:00 A.M. coffee break, and two more at lunch would add up to 750 milligrams.

But the brain isn't the only organ to get thrown for a loop by too much caffeine. Heart, lungs, stomach, bladder, kidneys, and pancreas can also get
40   confused because, just like the brain, caffeine keeps these organs falsely stimu-

lated. The heart and respiratory systems respond by quickening their pace, which can raise blood pressure and shorten breath. The stomach responds by overproducing potentially harmful stomach acids—a precursor of ulcers. And the kidneys and bladder find themselves working overtime in the bathroom. Coffee's pharmacological effects add up to something of an Indianapolis 500 for the entire body.

Which is fine for those of us with the sense to take appropriate pit stops. Those of us hooked on coffee, however, make the mistake of keeping our systems racing constantly. As one cup begins to wear off, we reach for another —the result of which can be sleeplessness, irritability, tremors, and fatigue as the body never quiets down to the point of getting the rest it needs. The consequences of this perpetual joyride can be less than joyful.

For anyone with a history of heart trouble, coffee's fun and games *could* be fatal. A number of studies have gone so far as to indict coffee as a cause of heart attacks in the population at large, but these surveys have thus far fallen short of the evidence needed for a guilty verdict. People who are already "coronary prone" are the only ones who really need to worry—yet this category is broader than you might think. If you suffer from angina, high blood pressure, or diabetes, consider yourself a member.

People with other existing problems also need to avoid coffee, decaffeinated brands included. (It's not the caffeine but rather a combination of other chemicals present in the coffee bean that stimulates the stomach to produce excess acids.) With ulcers, worry itself seems to be as hard on the stomach as anything we put into it. So if you *do* enjoy an occasional cup of coffee, do yourself the favor of at least not letting it bother you.

Coffee's primary danger for most of us seems to be, quite simply, that it's a convenient, relatively inexpensive, and *accepted* way of putting our bodies into a state of excitement that can be addictive—*and* potentially counterproductive. My own experience with coffee is that I know I've had too much when I start making lists that I only lose.

So treat coffee as you would alcohol—with respect. And be aware that coffee is not the only source of caffeine (see following table). Remember, something in the neighborhood of 250 milligrams of caffeine a day ought to be your limit. Anything substantially beyond that and you invite the very ineffectiveness you're trying to correct.

Remember, too, that there are other ways of staying alert. Caffeine works its magic by making your heart beat faster and increasing your body's output of adrenaline—but then so does exercise. So how about some quick jumping jacks or a little running in place to stave off those drooping eyelids. Splash those lids with some cold water after you've gotten them a little sweaty and you'll really feel rejuvenated.

If you're afraid you'll miss the warmth and aroma of that steaming eight-ounce crutch, keep in mind that herbal teas and broths can be every bit as flavorful.

Caffeine: It's Not Only in Coffee

	Caffeine* (milligrams)
Coffee (6 ounces)	
Brewed:	
Maxwell House, electric perk	97
Folgers Vacuum Packed, electric perk	90
Hills Brothers, ground	90
Yuban, electric perk	75
Instant:	
Hills Brothers	80
Folgers Crystals	75
Kava	53–75
Maxwell House	57
Nescafe	56
Taster's Choice, freeze-dried	56
Maxim, freeze-dried	55
Yuban	50
Decaffeinated types	2–5
Coffee blends:	
Luzianne Premium, ground	66
Sunrise, instant	52
Mellow Roast, ground	48
Tea (6 ounces)	
Brewed:	
English Breakfast	78
Red Rose	62
Salada	60
Lipton	53
Tetley	48
Instant:	
Lipton	(NA)
Nestea	(NA)
Soft Drink (12 ounces)	
Mountain Dew	49
Tab	45
Coca-Cola	42
Dr. Pepper	40
RC Cola	36

	Caffeine* (milligrams)
Soft Drink (*continued*)	
Pepsi-Cola	35
Diet Pepsi	34
Pepsi Light	34
RC 100	0
Medication (1 tablet)	
Stimulants:	
Vivarin	200
Nodoz	100
Weight control:	
Dexatrim	200
Appedrine	100
Painkillers:	
Excedrin	64.8
Vanquish	33
Anacin	32.5
Bromo-Seltzer (1 capful)	32.5
Empirin Compound	32.2
Empirin	0
Cold and allergy drugs:	
Sinarest	30
Dristan	16.2
Menstrual aids:	
Pre-Mens Forte	100
Femicin	65
Midol	32.4

NOTES: *Per portion of beverage or medication cited.
NA—information not available.

SOURCES: Information supplied by companies. Values also adapted from *Handbook of Non-Prescription Drugs*, 5th ed. (Washington, D.C.: American Pharmaceutical Association, 1977); and "A Study of Caffeine in Tea," by Daniel S. Grosser (*American Journal of Clinical Nutrition*, October, 1978).

The word to remember with coffee, as with life's other pleasures, is moderation. Enjoyed judiciously, it can be a relatively harmless boost. It is *not*, however, something to be relied upon. Play the seesaw game of alternating highs and lows long enough, and you may find that coffee will lose its elevating effects altogether. And then where would you be? Left with the lows and the lows only.

10/

Cigarettes: The Riskiest Vice of All, but There Are Ways of Improving the Odds

Rather than burden you with a depressing array of statistics, we'll make an analogy, short and sour: If immoderate drinking and being obese could be likened to playing Russian roulette with one bullet, smoking could be likened to playing with two. Smokers of a pack or more of cigarettes a day are two times as likely to die from lung cancer, bronchitis, emphysema, or heart disease—and chop as much as nine years off their lives as a result. Smoking is every bit the health hazard that the government keeps telling it is.

So why do one in three adults continue to do it?

The obvious answer, and one in keeping with the philosophy of this book, would be because smoking affords pleasure. But how pleasurable can something be, really, when its dangers stare us so directly in the face?

No, pleasure may be part of the reason people smoke, but not as large a part as addiction. Nicotine has been called a more addicting drug than heroin. A study done in England showed that 85 percent of all teenagers who smoked more than one cigarette in their lives went on to get hooked. Soldiers in prisoner of war camps during World War I are reported to have bartered food for tobacco even when rations fell below 900 calories a day.

"People will tell you that smoking calms them, that it helps them work, that it does positive things for them. And that that's why they smoke," says Stanley Schachter, Ph.D., a psychologist from Columbia University. "What these people fail to reveal, however, is that they climb walls when they can't [smoke]."

Indeed, it is the curse of addicting drugs that—more than making us feel good when we take them—they make us feel rotten when we don't. And nicotine qualifies. The guy who used to walk that mile for a Camel wasn't out for exercise.

So nicotine is seriously addictive. The rest of the bad news is that the way we most commonly get nicotine—through cigarettes—is noxious. As equipped as our respiratory systems are for dealing with a certain amount of pollutants

44

in the air, they are *not* equipped to handle the repeated and concentrated barrage that inhaling cigarette smoke inflicts. The combination of heat and tar in cigarette smoke has a paralyzing effect on the lung's tiny hairlike filtering devices called cilia. As soon as these cilia become less active, our lungs become all the more susceptible to future abuse, be it in the form of more cigarette smoke or simply the chemical *and bacterial* pollutants we face every day. Smoking, in short, takes away the lungs' protective devices while at the same time it takes potentially cancer-causing jabs at the sensitive lung tissue that these devices were designed to protect.

But that's not all smoking does: It adversely affects our hearts, our stomachs, our mental faculties, even our sexuality. Let's look at the heart.

It may seem strange that putting something into your lungs can be detrimental to your heart, but it can. Heart disease, first of all, is actually something of a misnomer because it's our blood vessels, not our hearts, that usually get sick. The heart is the one to suffer ultimately, of course, but an estimated 80 percent of all heart problems get their start—and owe their finish—to a gradual clogging of arteries and veins called atherosclerosis. Factors other than smoking can contribute to this process (dietary fats, high blood pressure, and inactivity, for example) but cigarette smoking may be the worst offender of all because it attacks the circulatory system in several different ways at the same time.

The nicotine in cigarette smoke (having entered the blood via the lungs) damages tiny particles in the blood called platelets, which in turn become "trash," a likely forerunner of (or contributor to) the buildup of atherosclerotic plaque inside artery walls.

Nicotine also stimulates the production of chemical substances called catecholamines, which are known to increase heart rate, blood pressure, and the oxygen needs of the heart. These effects may have serious consequences in a heart already short of adequate nourishment because blood vessels are being narrowed by nicotine-induced plaque.

Then, too, smoking infuses the blood with inordinate amounts of carbon monoxide, reducing the blood's ability to transport oxygen and thickening it, thus encouraging *clotting* in arteries narrowed by plaque.

Cigarette smoking, in short, increases the heart's needs at the same time it decreases its supplies. It's a bad situation, one that may increase by sixfold a heavy smoker's risk of heart attack over a nonsmoker's.

As for cigarettes' effects on the stomach, the danger here lies with ulcers. Nicotine tends to reduce the bicarbonate output of the pancreas, thus creating the kind of acidic conditions on which ulcers thrive.

Smoking's effects on the brain? As alert as you may *think* your cigarettes are making you, a study done at the University of California at Los Angeles showed that tobacco smoke *impaired* both short- and long-term memory (*American Journal of Psychiatry,* February, 1978).

Smoking and sex?

Cigarettes may look sexy, but that, unfortunately, is where the connection ends. Heavy smoking in men has been shown to reduce testosterone (male hormone) levels and also contribute to the immobilization and destruction of sperm. And in pregnant women who smoke, it's been shown that many of smoking's ill effects get passed on to baby. Toss in the fact that smoking gives both sexes bad breath and it's a wonder cigarettes ever got mixed up with sex appeal to begin with.

If all this makes you want to quit, or cut down, or be glad that you *have* quit, or thankful that you never took up smoking in the first place, that's good. Because of all the vices out there, smoking is one that we can't think of a single thing to say something nice about. That smoking can help you keep your weight down? One way of looking at that is that it's doing so by keeping you sickly. Virtually every bodily function, either directly or indirectly, is adversely affected by smoking cigarettes.

But there is hope. And we don't mean in the form of a cure for lung cancer. For one, there are ways of reducing your desire to smoke by eating certain *healthful* foods; there are also ways of making the smoking you *do* give in to less harmful by fortifying yourself with certain vitamins.

A Diet to Help You Quit Smoking

It's been shown that the more acidic your body's chemical balance, the faster you flush nicotine out of your system. So the trick is to eat foods that are alkaline, say James Fix, Ph.D., and David M. Daughton, two psychologists from the University of Nebraska College of Medicine. The more alkaline you are, they theorize, the less you should need to smoke in order to maintain a level of nicotine in your blood with which you can feel comfortable.

They got their idea from Dr. Schachter, who contends that you smoke for the nicotine you get—not for something to do with your hands—and that stress, alcohol, and acidic foods can drain you of your supply. He found that students under stress, for example, had highly acidic urine, and that people geared up at parties had the same.

Was it the anxiety that was making them smoke more? Or was it the acidic chemistry that this anxiety was producing? Dr. Schachter gave the students highly alkaline bicarbonate of soda to find out—and sure enough, as acid levels were reduced, so was smoking.

It's also why people tend to smoke more in the morning, he says, since the body is more acidic after it has slept.

"Any kind of physiological factor can be important in determining smoking behavior," says Brett Silverstein, Ph.D., a colleague of Dr. Schachter. Experiments with teenagers, for example, have shown that those with acidic urine—females, especially—were more apt to smoke than a group that was alkaline. And after a five-week group therapy session designed to help adults quit the habit, it was discovered that 82 percent of those who had failed were "acidic."

How can diet help?

You are what you eat, so by restricting yourself to foods that are alkaline, you should be able to control your body chemistry and hence your appetite for nicotine.

Concerned about gaining weight if you quit?

Don't be. Most highly alkaline foods are low in calories—and good for you. (Just take a look at the accompanying table.) The best alkalizers are vegetables; the worst are meat and alcohol. Keep that in mind the next time you're offered those little sausages wrapped in bacon at a cocktail party.

Some Foods to Help You Quit Smoking

	Portion	Alkalizing Effect	Calories
Molasses	2 teaspoons	+60.0	40
Raisins	⅓ cup	+34.0	131
Figs, dried	1½	+33.0	83
Lima beans, green	⅔ cup	+28.0	125
Spinach	1 cup	+27.0	22
Kidney beans	⅔ cup	+18.0	88
Brewer's yeast	1 tablespoon	+17.1	35
Soybeans, green	⅔ cup	+17.0	158
Bean sprouts	1 cup	+16.0	66
Almonds	12	+12.0	88
Brussels sprouts	6	+11.0	53
Carrot	1 large	+11.0	40
Cucumber	10 slices	+ 7.9	7
Celery	2 stalks	+ 7.8	8
Lettuce	¼ head	+ 7.4	12
Grapefruit juice	½ cup	+ 7.0	75
Potato	1	+ 7.0	101
Pineapple	2 slices	+ 6.8	57
Peach	1 large	+ 5.9	49
Banana	1 small	+ 5.6	96
Orange juice	½ cup	+ 5.6	48
Tomato	1 small	+ 5.6	20
Strawberries	12	+ 5.5	36
Mushrooms	7	+ 4.0	30
Apple	1 large	+ 3.7	90
Milk, whole	7 ounces	+ 2.3	145
Onion	1	+ 1.5	23

NOTE: Values are given for foods in the raw state.

SOURCE: Adapted from *Hawk's Physiological Chemistry,* edited by Bernard L. Oser (New York: McGraw-Hill, 1965).

Now for some vitamin therapy.

The human lung, as we said, is equipped with cilia, tiny hairlike projections designed to undulate in a way that escorts foreign matter back up and out of the lungs in the form of mucus or phlegm. Smoking, though, tends to paralyze these cilia, giving germs and potentially cancer-causing agents free access to the deeper, more sensitive areas of the lung. It's important to keep these cilia active, and research done at the Delta Regional Primate Research Center at Tulane University suggests that vitamin A can do that.

James C. S. Kim, D.V.M., Sc.D., several years ago exposed three groups of hamsters to badly polluted air five hours a week for eight weeks. The conditions, he said, were "comparable not only to industrial pollution found in an urban-suburban environment, but also to the exposure of the respiratory system of a habitual smoker."

The first group was fed a diet lacking in vitamin A; the second, what Dr. Kim called a diet "adequate" in A; and the third, a menu "high" in the nutrient.

How did they hold up?

The hamsters deficient in A displayed "rapid and often labored breathing" during their exposures, and by the fifth week of the experiment, Dr. Kim said, their health had "visibly started to decline."

The hamsters adequate and high in A, on the other hand, showed a somewhat increased rate of breathing, but no other signs of distress and remained in good condition throughout the eight weeks of the experiment.

When the lungs of these animals were examined under a microscope, the A-deficient group showed severe damage. Epithelial lining had degenerated; cilia, necessary for defense against bacteria, had been either seriously impaired or destroyed; and cells in the alveoli (the little sacs which permit oxygen to pass from the air into the bloodstream) had hardened. Many of the hamsters showed signs of pneumonia. And abnormal cell growth—the kind that can lead to cancer—was widespread.

The A-adequate groups, by comparison, showed far less damage. The pollutants had left a mark, but epithelial linings were intact. There were no signs of pneumonia, and abnormal cell growth was minimal.

Then there was the five-year study of 8,278 Norwegian men conducted by E. Bjelke, Ph.D., in 1975 in which it was discovered that clients high in vitamin A were responsible for lower lung cancer rates in all age groups, smokers included.

These discoveries merit the attention of more than just smokers, however. All of us have to breathe air that is not as pure as we would like, and vitamin A appears to aid in the regeneration of lung tissue in a way that can help us do that more healthfully.

What are the best sources of vitamin A? Vegetables, luckily—the very foods that can reduce the desire to smoke in the first place. The RDA for vitamin A is 5,000 international units (I.U.) for adult men (about 4,000 I.U.

Foods High in Vitamin A

	Portion	Vitamin A (I.U.)
Liver, cooked	3 ounces	45,390
Sweet potato, cooked	1 medium	11,940
Carrots, cooked	½ cup	8,140
Spinach, cooked	½ cup	7,290
Cantaloupe	¼ medium	4,620
Kale, cooked	½ cup	4,565
Broccoli, cooked	1 medium stalk	4,500
Winter squash, cooked	½ cup	4,305
Mustard greens, cooked	½ cup	4,060
Apricots, fresh	3 medium	2,890
Watermelon	10″ × 1″ slice	2,510
Endive	1 cup	1,650
Leaf lettuce	1 cup	1,050
Asparagus, cooked	4 medium	540
Peas, cooked	½ cup	430
Green beans, cooked	½ cup	340
Yellow corn, cooked	½ cup	330
Parsley, dried	1 tablespoon	303
Egg, hard-cooked	1 large	260

NOTE: I.U.—international units.

SOURCES: Adapted from U.S. Department of Agriculture Handbook nos. 8-1, 8-2, and 456.

for adult women) and you get 16,280 of those in just one cup of cooked carrots. Spinach, broccoli, winter squash, and sweet potatoes are also very high, as is liver. Vitamin A supplements are available, but because too much vitamin A (over 100,000 I.U.) can be toxic, it would be our suggestion that you get your A from the foods listed in the accompanying table.

Vitamin C is the second vitamin that smokers should get in abundance. Smoking depletes the body of vitamin C (to the tune of about 25 milligrams per cigarette), and vitamin C appears to be important for the proper functioning of the body's immune system, a system which smoking, as we've shown, can already burden heavily.

How much vitamin C should smokers get?

As much as it takes to put their minds at ease. C is one vitamin where the more seems to be the merrier. There are no dangers of overdose with C; doctors have used, with no ill effects, amounts as high as 10 grams daily to treat a variety of disorders.

Vitamin C supplementation is well worth considering; this does not mean, however, that natural sources should be overlooked. As with vitamin A, many

Foods High in Vitamin C

	Portion	Vitamin C (milligrams)
Orange juice, fresh-squeezed	1 cup	124
Green pepper	½ cup	96
Grapefruit juice	1 cup	93
Papaya	½	85
Brussels sprouts, cooked	4	73
Broccoli	½ cup	70
Orange	1 medium	66
Turnip greens, cooked	½ cup	50
Cantaloupe	¼ medium	45
Cauliflower	½ cup	45
Strawberries	½ cup	44
Tomato juice	1 cup	39
Grapefruit	½	37
Potato, baked	1 medium	31
Tomato	1 medium	28
Cabbage	½ cup	21
Blackberries	½ cup	15
Spinach	½ cup	14
Blueberries	½ cup	10
Cherries, sweet	½ cup	8
Mung bean sprouts	¼ cup	5

SOURCE: U.S. Department of Agriculture Handbook no. 456.

foods high in C are also good for reducing the body's acidity and hence, as the theory goes, the desire to smoke in the first place.

As negative as this chapter has been, I don't think I've treated smoking unfairly. Because unless you've got yourself to the point where you smoke only when you really enjoy it, smoking is *not* the great source of pleasure that this country's acres of billboards would have us believe. It's something that—once addicted—we do just to "break even." And how much fun can that be?

I've seen too many people feel too good when they quit, and too many people look too pasty gray when they don't. At least alcohol bestows a flush.

If you've tried to quit but have failed, why not at least cut down? The dangers of smoking are very much dose-related: The more you do, the more you risk—right down to the puff. So select your puffs more wisely. Allow yourself a certain number of cigarettes a day and concentrate on enjoying them. You may even find that by smoking less, you enjoy it more. Isn't it, after all, the cigarette that you've missed most that you enjoy most? So miss a few more. Feel as though you've earned your couple of smokes a day and they're liable to provide as much pleasure as the pack that's now only got you coughing and feeling guilty.

As for the advantages of switching to a low-tar brand, they're mixed. Studies show that the low-tar brands are helping to reduce cases of lung cancer, but heart disease doesn't seem to be enjoying similar benefits.

Why? Converts to low-tar brands tend to inhale the things down to their toes in order to reap the kicks they're used to, and that means they suck in as much—if not more—carbon monoxide than when they smoke the higher-tar brands. And it's carbon monoxide that is the main culprit in heart disease.

There are plenty of programs you can join to help you control your smoking, and most of them are very good. But your own program can be very good, too. Maybe even better. Because no one, after all, knows more about your smoking than you do.

11/

Stress: Learn How to Handle It and It Can Keep You Healthy

There's been a lot of talk about stress lately. Too much, I think, because the talk itself has created stress. There's a study out now telling us that even Christmas is stressful. Now *that's* stressful.

No, with a little less talk—and a little more action—we could take a good deal of the starch out of stress, and I'm not alone in believing that.

"It's not the amount of stress you have so much as it is how you handle it," says 74-year-old Hans Selye, M.D., Ph.D., Nobel laureate and president of the International Institute of Stress in Montreal. Which is maybe why some of us can live to be president of the United States at age 70 without so much as a gray hair to show for it, while others die of heart attacks in our forties just trying to sell shoes. We each have our own ways of dealing with stress, and some of us, clearly, are better at it than others.

Why?

Before we get into that, let's take a closer look at what stress is. We throw the word around so much, we rarely stop to analyze what it is we're throwing.

"There are two kinds of stress: short-term and long-term," says stress expert Kenneth R. Pelletier, Ph.D., a clinical psychologist and author of numerous books on the subject. "Short-term stress [basic survival stuff, like getting out of the way of a bus] we can take; it's the long-term kind [like having to balance unbalanceable checkbooks] that gives us trouble." And the reason it gives us trouble is that it never lets up.

When a stress can be immediately resolved, Dr. Pelletier explains, it can actually be good for us. The biochemical events that are involved in successfully sidestepping that bus, for example, are evolutionarily established responses that can actually leave us feeling more alive—as you may have noticed.

Long-term stresses, however, have no such rejuvenating effect. On the contrary, they can wear us down both physically and emotionally because they offer no relief. When we suspect that the checkbook that doesn't balance this week isn't going to balance next week either, our bodies remain in a state of semiarousal, a lesser version of what we experience for the brief moments we're in the path of that bus. And when this state of semiarousal persists for too long,

Learn to Break Up Stress and It Won't Break You

Short-Term Stress: The Healthy Kind

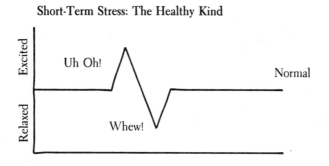

Long-Term Stress: The Hazardous Kind

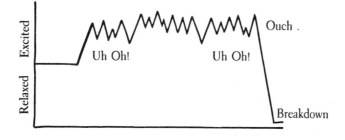

The Even Keel

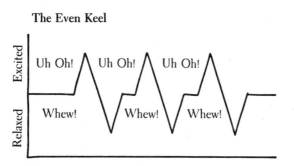

For every "uh oh," in other words, you had better find a "whew."

we quite literally can begin to come apart at the seams. Heart disease, cancer, high blood pressure, emotional breakdowns, obesity, hemorrhoids, headaches, alcoholism, drug abuse—all have been linked to the biological consequences of living under constant pressure.

So how do we deal with long-term stresses?

We'd like to be able to say by resolving them, but as we all know, balanced checkbooks are easier said than done. So the next best approach, Dr. Pelletier says, is to learn to break up chronic stress patterns, even if it takes some practice to do it. Exercise, a relaxing hobby, the enjoyment of art, . . . anything that allows the mind and/or body a moment of reprieve has potential for releasing some of the tension that chronic stress accumulates.

Dr. Pelletier sees these periodic moments of reprieve as paralleling—and being as important as—the periods of rest that the heart takes between beats. To endure we must, as the heart does, refurbish ourselves at regular intervals or we risk burning out.

Perhaps even more importantly, though, as we learn to relax and take the time to improve our health, we begin to feel better about ourselves in ways that help us deal with stress in the first place. And *that's* where the real benefit of stress reduction lies.

"It's really as much of a conceptual shift as anything else," Dr. Pelletier notes. "When people begin to pay attention to their health, they seem to have a much better ability to look at things that used to bug them and simply [to be more detached]. If you're taking time out of your life to exercise, for example, you're taking a psychological stance that *in itself* is going to have you reacting differently to your job, your office, your sense of achievement, your career."

Staying healthy, in other words, can give us the emotional as well as the physical strength to stand up to the nonstop pressures of modern-day life. And the people who are managing to deal with stress most effectively are doing just that: staying healthy. Ronald Reagan rides horses. Jimmy Carter jogged. Very few presidents have neglected their health, perhaps for the simple reason that they can't afford to.

So yes, you can sit on the edge of your chair and read about how next Christmas is going to give you a heart attack . . . or you can get up, exercise, eat right, teach yourself how to relax, and enjoy playing Santa Claus for quite a few more years. Stress can be a killer, or it can be one of the best health motivators of all.

Your Job—Love It or Leave It

They rant, they rave. They pull at their hair until everything is perfect. And yet musical conductors, despite the hazards of their trade, manage to outlive the rest of us by an average of eight years.

How? By loving their work.

"Without work, all life goes rotten," said Albert Camus. "But when work is without soul, life stifles and dies." Maestros have soul.

"Blocking the fulfillment of our natural drives for any great period of time can be a very dangerous thing," says Hans Selye, M.D., Ph.D.

Which could explain why high-level management lives longer than mid-level. Frustration is what kills. And the bored die sooner than the busy.

"Stress is an inescapable part of life," according to Dr. Selye. "The idea is to get it to work *for* rather than against us."

How? "By committing ourselves to serving a cause we can respect." We are at heart more "moral," says Dr. Selye, than many of us may care to admit.

If all this sounds like a little too much philosophical hogwash, note, if you will, the conclusion reached several years ago by a special task force commissioned by the federal government to study the life spans of this country's labor force. "More so than any measure of physical health, the use of tobacco, or genetic inheritance," the report states, "the number one predictor of longevity in this country is work satisfaction."

You might keep that in mind the next time you go to kick the copy machine.

12/

It's Okay to Be a Workaholic If . . .

Up until about a hundred years ago there was no such thing as a "workaholic." Because not until the Industrial Revolution came along and established "hours" was there the possibility of working too many of them. Sure, Sundays were off limits. But that still left Monday through Saturday to work as hard and as long as we darn well pleased.

So what happens now when we try to put in a couple of 14-hour days back to back? Family, family physician, peers—even the janitor—tell us to slow down.

Is it really so bad to work hard? Is it unhealthy?

Yes and no to both of those questions. Work, like alcohol, is bad and unhealthy only if it produces bad and unhealthy results. If what you're doing is causing trauma, either to you or to someone else, then it's certainly not good and probably not healthy. But if your routine is stepping on no one's toes but your own—and you rather enjoy the pain—then there's very little scientific data to argue you've got a problem.

"We hear a great deal these days about the dangers of overwork and excessive striving, and of being the so-called Type A personality. But I think that in many ways this is exaggerated and arouses unnecessary anxiety," says Hans Selye, M.D., Ph.D.

Marilyn Machlowitz, Ph.D., seconds that opinion. She believes that the stress many workaholics feel comes from *outside* rather than from within. "It is often the familial and societal pressures to conform to the norm that create conflict, guilt, and stress—not the work itself," she writes in her book *Workaholics: Living with Them, Working with Them* (Addison-Wesley, 1980).

We had an opportunity to speak with Dr. Machlowitz (a confessed workaholic herself) by phone (she was nice enough to make time for us during her dinner hour), and she explained (as she dried dishes) that most of the work addicts she talked to were in fact very happy, successful, and well-adjusted people. "They were in jobs that they were very good at and enjoyed immensely," she said.

There is, however, another side to the workaholic story—the side seen by

New York City psychiatrist Jay B. Rohrlich, M.D., every day in his practice.

"The workaholics I see are not happy people," Dr. Rohrlich told us. "They are using work to block out emotional disorders or to fulfill neurotic needs."

He adds, "There is no typical work addict because each finds something different about work that he or she finds gratifying. Some like the aggressiveness they can display in the work environment. Others crave the security and order their work provides. Some enjoy the competitive aspects of work. There are even some who become addicted to the comforts of being in a subservient role in the workplace."

In his book *Work and Love: The Crucial Balance* (Summit Books, 1980), Dr. Rohrlich divides work addicts into ten major categories. We have done our best to condense these descriptions, as follows:

- *the hostile work addict,* who attacks work instead of some person or situation he has come to resent.
- *the ashamed work addict,* who prefers the image he projects at work to the one he is saddled with at home.
- *the competitive work addict,* for whom the work environment is an arena in which to keep score.
- *the defensive work addict,* who uses work to keep his mind off painful emotions.
- *the friendless work addict,* for whom the work environment provides a sense of belonging.
- *the guilty work addict,* whose long hours are a form of self-punishment.
- *the latent homosexual work addict,* who enjoys being controlled by bosses or clients.
- *the obsessive work addict,* for whom work satisfies a neurotic need for neatness and order.
- *the pre- or post-psychotic work addict,* who can maintain no sense of self outside the work structure.
- *the sexually frustrated or impotent work addict,* for whom work provides a chance to flirt in ways that need never face a test of consummation.

Many of those categories overlap, Dr. Rohrlich says, but they provide a fairly clear view of the basic types of work addiction, nonetheless. Not a very pretty picture.

But then, as a psychiatrist, Dr. Rohrlich sees only those workaholics for whom work has become a problem. The workaholics interviewed by Dr. Machlowitz gave her cause to categorize workaholism in a different light entirely. If people like Dick Vermeil, Jessica Savitch, William Proxmire, Barbara Walters, and Neil Simon have psychological problems we should all be so lucky. After interviewing more than 100 such functional work addicts, Dr. Machlowitz classified them as:

- *the dedicated workaholic,* totally without outside interests and proud of it. "I'm so single-minded I have to work very hard at not working 24 hours a day," offered one.
- *the integrated workaholic,* lucky enough to have a job so enjoyably diverse that *not* working seems like a chore. As David Rockefeller, chairman of Chase Manhattan Bank, once told the *New Yorker,* "I can't imagine a more interesting job than mine. . . . There is no field of activity it isn't involved in."
- *the diffuse workaholic,* who has his hands in everything—good on the job, but even better at serving on community boards, coaching Little League, rebuilding antique cars, and writing memoirs. "These people may change jobs and fields fairly frequently," Dr. Machlowitz notes.
- *the intense workaholic,* who attacks leisure with the same fervor as work. "More than one person in my sample was a marathoner," she told us, "applying the same energy to their racing as to their careers."

So there you have it: the two sides of the workaholic story. A little like the light and dark side of the moon, it would seem, though in reality the good and bad are not so distinct.

Even workaholics in need of help, Dr. Rohrlich says, have great strengths: indomitable energy and sense of commitment, misdirected though they may be. And many of the successful work addicts studied by Dr. Machlowitz had their shortcomings: brusqueness, egocentricity, intolerance, and inflexibility—all of which, believe it or not, can wind up costing the workaholic some of the efficiency he worships.

One M.D., in fact, asserts that the notion of the workaholic being efficient is a myth. "It takes him 12 hours to do what others can do in only 8." Often he is reluctant to delegate authority; or he will have a compulsive need for things to be perfect; or he will tend to pursue things that interest him rather than things that are of importance. All these behaviors can wind up seriously undermining effectiveness. When work is all one has, inefficiency can be very industrious at disguising itself.

This seems to be the bottom line on work abuse in general. If you can honestly say that working long hours is—in all ways—really *working,* then keep it up. But if your hard work is, in fact, becoming an easy way out, if it's helping you avoid your family and yourself, if it's blunting your sensitivities to life's other pleasures . . . we challenge you to try a more leisurely schedule.

Are You a Workaholic?

In her book *Workaholics,* Marilyn Machlowitz, Ph.D., has compiled the following questions to help you find out. Answer yes to eight or more, she says, and your chances look pretty good.

1. Do you get up early, no matter how late you go to bed?
2. If you're eating lunch alone, do you read or work while you eat?
3. Do you make daily lists of things to do?
4. Do you find it difficult to "do nothing"?
5. Are you energetic and competitive?
6. Do you work on weekends and holidays?
7. Can you work anytime and anywhere?
8. Do you find vacations "hard to take"?
9. Do you dread retirement?
10. Do you really enjoy your work?

SOURCE: Excerpted from *Workaholics: Living with Them, Working with Them,* by Marilyn Machlowitz. Copyright 1980 by Marilyn Machlowitz. Reprinted with permission of Addison-Wesley Publishing Co.

13/

How and Why to Cut Down
on Blowing Up

Somehow we've come to consider it healthy and natural to blow our stacks. "Lets off steam," as we like to say. That notion deserves a second look.

If abused, stack-blowing should be considered a bad habit the same as cigarettes, alcohol, junk food, and drugs. It is *not* good for us. And it may not even be all that natural. After all . . .

What, for the thousands of years we roamed the earth in our loin cloths, was there to get violently angry about? Scared, maybe. And frustrated, as our last spear would miss its mark. But angry? Probably not very often. Anger happens when we feel wronged. And for the thousands of years that survival was our main concern, we had to contend first and foremost with Mother Nature, who does not do *wrong*, but rather only does things that we might not always *like* her to do. It's people who do wrong. And credit unions. And only relatively recently have we had to deal at any great length with either of those.

No, we would all do well to stop considering it so healthy and natural to blow our stacks because blowing our stacks, first of all, probably means that we're warehousing more "steam" than we should. Worse yet, if you get angry a lot, chances are you're wrong a lot—and how healthy can that be? By the simple law of averages, not all Sunday drivers, waiters, secretaries, and report cards can be as bad as you make them out to be. If you get angry a lot, chances are you're out of touch—with yourself and with your environment. You feel wronged because you have a wrong idea of what you have a right to expect. And that, because it's stressful, can be unhealthful.

Anger is a "form of energy which if repressed . . can harm almost any part of the body," says Leo Madow, M.D., in his book *Anger: How to Recognize and Cope with It* (Charles Scribner's Sons, 1972). Headaches, ulcers, bowel problems, respiratory ills, skin flareups, arthritis, high blood pressure, heart attacks, and a variety of mental disorders can be the result of keeping anger bottled up. (See following box.)

But blowing your stack isn't the answer either, since that approach only leaves you having to put back together a lot of bruised pieces.

60

No, you're best off treating anger with respect. Because when you reserve anger for rare occasions, it takes on a noble rather than a neurotic air. It shows that instead of being out of touch with reality, you are acutely *aware* of reality. It demonstrates that you have a firm sense of justice, and courage to defend it.

Which all sounds fine until you get down to some real-life situations—like coming home to cold spaghetti and a D from Junior in geometry after a miserable day at work. That's when noble restraint gets hard to come by, and harsh words come easily.

"There are no simple solutions to the problems of anger and no pat formulas for dealing with the complex issues often involved," Dr. Madow warns. That does *not* mean, however, that it cannot be controlled.

He outlines four basic steps to help keep anger at bay. To these four we have added a fifth: fitness. After reading his suggestions, we think you'll see why.

First off, Dr. Madow says, learn to recognize your anger. That may sound simple enough, but in all too many cases it is not. "Anger may be denied because we feel too guilty about it, or are afraid of it," he points out. It may be easier to make light of our anger in the form of sarcasm. Or we may wind up feeling depressed by it, or sleepless and tense. Anger can disguise itself in a number of forms.

Once you've decided you *are* angry, the next step, he says, is to determine *at what.* Your boss? That can present problems, so you probably grouch at your family instead. It can be difficult to ferret out the real instigators of anger, Dr. Madow says—and sometimes dangerous. But it has to be done before peace can be made.

Step three is figuring out *why* you're angry. And that can be difficult, too, says Dr. Madow, because many times it becomes apparent that you have no reason to be. "We often experience anger because we have taken as personal something that may not be personal at all." Junior's D in geometry. The driver who thinks every day is Sunday.

And finally he stresses the importance of dealing with anger *realistically.* But once you've established the existence, the source, and the cause of your anger, that should be easy. No sense in upending a perfectly good plate of cold spaghetti when it's the chairman of the board that you'd really like to turn upside down.

Dealing with anger, as you can see, necessitates compromise. Which is what the process of "growing up" is all about. As infants—because our needs were simple—we could have what we wanted when we wanted it. But as our needs became gradually more complicated, so did the processes by which we procured them.

"Growing up consists of increasing limitation of direct, immediate satisfaction of needs," Dr. Madow says. As adults we must learn to live with other people's needs as well as our own. We must learn to accept responsibilities that

(*continued on page 64*)

Why It's Best to "Discuss It" . . .

You can do one of three things when you feel angry: You can sit tight and wait for the storm to pass; you can blow your stack; or you can . . . "discuss it."

Researchers at the University of Michigan looked into the relative merits of each of these approaches, and found that discussing it beat the other two maneuvers hands down. What they measured in coming to this conclusion was that all-important barometer of psychic turmoil we call blood pressure. The study's principal investigator, Ernest Harburg, Ph.D., talked about the results:

"Confronted with hostility, people usually explode in anger, bottle it up, or take steps to resolve the conflict. We found that people who remained relatively calm when confronted with conflict had lower than expected blood pressures. A typical response used by these people was, 'Let's be cool, let's deal with the problem!' "

The University of Michigan study focused on two groups of people: those living in high-stress areas (characterized by high crime and unemployment rates) and those living in low-stress areas (characterized by low crime and low unemployment rates). And in both groups, it was discovered that people who bottled up anger had the highest blood pressures; those who became openly hostile had the second highest readings; and those who took action to resolve their anger had the lowest.

Dr. Harburg described the discuss-it approach as "a way in which you explore the problem in a detached manner. You acknowledge your anger, but you are not openly hostile, verbally or physically, to the other person. Discussion involves detachment, reflection, conversation, and a willingness to solve the problem." The approach works, he feels, because it removes the cause of anger.

Interestingly, Dr. Harburg's study found that white collar workers use the discuss-it approach more than blue collar folks, and women use it more than men.

And Bad to Bottle It Up

Perhaps only fear has the ability to generate as much physical energy as anger. We slam doors, shout obscenities, maybe even punch each other in the mouth. But what happens when we don't?

This energy must go somewhere, and it does: It slams doors and shouts obscenities inside us.

When we get angry, our bodies prepare for action, and a number of internal changes take place: blood sugar gets mobilized for increased energy; blood pressure goes up; the heart beats faster to supply extra nourishment; adrenaline is secreted to dilate the pupils of the eyes to help us see better and to excite other senses.

Which is fine as long as we can totally purge ourselves of these emergency preparations. But in a civilized world, too often we cannot.

"If there is no discharge of this buildup, as is usually the case, we remain in a constant state of preparedness . . . and eventually this condition can harm us physically," says Leo Madow, M.D. He goes on to explain how.

Headaches: "Although there are many known organic causes of headache, by far the most common cause is tension. And tension is probably most often created by repressed anger. The tension headache is often described as a feeling of a very tight skullcap or a band around the head. The pains frequently go down the back of the neck and are sometimes attributed to muscle disease or a pinched nerve, but probably the [most common] cause is muscle tension resulting from accumulated hidden anger."

Ulcers: The person who develops an ulcer from emotional causes is one who is basically dependent and wants to be mothered, Dr. Madow says. "However, he cannot tolerate these dependency wishes and becomes angry at himself. This anger is probably one of the essential factors in the development of ulcers." It causes increased blood flow and greater than normal secretions of acids in the stomach.

High blood pressure: When there is a perpetual conflict between the desire to be aggressive and the obligation not to be (due either to fear, guilt, or wishes of approval), hypertension can be the result, because the circulatory system is being kept in a constant state of semipreparedness.

Dr. Madow also goes on to explain how repressed anger may lower our resistance to colds, contribute to itching and hives, exacerbate arthritis, make us impotent, cause depression, and even drive us to commit suicide. Evidence has also emerged that repressed anger may even increase chances of breast cancer in women. Virtually no corner of our bodies, evidently, is exempt from anger's ire, so we would do well to keep our cool.

we may not want to; we must learn to get along. And to do that, it helps to be happy—which is where fitness fits in.

Why It's Easier to Walk Softly When You're Fit

How many really fit people do you know with short fuses? Isn't it usually those of us who have let ourselves go who do most of the flying off the handle? There are reasons for that:

Self-esteem.   In order to remain calm when the chairman of the board falsely attributes a recent company failure to your department, it helps to be able to remain confident. And a lifestyle that you're proud of can help you do that.

A thinner waist.   It's amazing how much more we're apt to become dissatisfied with others when we're dissatisfied with ourselves. The simple job of commandeering a physique you're happy about can go a long way in keeping you in a frame of mind to look for the best in others.

Punishment.   Dr. Madow talks about the dangers of repressing anger due to feelings of guilt. So if you feel guilty for being angry that your parents never bought you a tricycle, go out and run a *hard* four miles. The nice thing about exercise is that it can be punishment, or it can be . . .

Reward.   Anger often builds because it gets fed by frustrations unrelated to its true source. People who have something they can regularly turn to for enjoyment, however—such as exercise—are much less apt to feel they're forever being cheated.

Escape.   The analogy of the caged rat here may be extreme, but appropriate nonetheless. Much anger stems from feelings of confinement (e.g., job, marriage, the responsibilities of parenthood). Exercise involves freedom of movement that has an uncanny way of giving these feelings room to breathe.

Humility.   If your short temper has its roots in a big head, what you may need is to find out how "little" your *body* is. Exercise has a way of keeping us in touch with our limitations.

Blissful fatigue.   Not that the true source of your anger should not be rousted out eventually, but there's nothing like sound relaxation to help you get your search party together. Exercise is a proven muscle relaxant. And tense muscles can affect your mind more than you may realize.

14/

Your Standard of Living: It's Not High If You're Hassled

Physical comfort is important—but not worth killing ourselves to get. Indeed, happiness is a delicate balance between material and spiritual reward. If you hate the job that's allowing you to drive your (temperamental) Porsche, if your peaceful home in the country necessitates a harrowing commute, if your swimming pool has you pulling your hair out in a losing battle against algae—how much comfort, really, can they be?

That's a question that a professor at the Indiana School of Business has designed a test to answer. "Income isn't everything," says Richard N. Farmer, Ph.D. "A living standard also depends on such factors as good health, quality schools, freedom from pollution, and other amenities."

In a word, satisfaction. And we agree. If your fat salary is earning you a fat stomach, chest pains, a drinking problem, and another divorce—how valuable, really, can it be?

"Considerations of this sort lead me to propose the 'Hassle Factor' as a microsocial measure for standards of living," Dr. Farmer says. His "Hassle Factor" is arrived at by way of a test, as we've said, which anyone can take to determine just how enviable his lot in life really is. We include the test at the end of this chapter, with hopes that it may afford you some healthful perspective on why you may be killing yourself to keep up payments on a car that's in the shop six months out of the year, anyway. The test: Dr. Farmer has identified 12 aspects of daily living that he feels are potential sources of hassle. By grading each (on a scale of 0 to 10), first in terms of its importance to you and then in terms of its quality, you come up with a numerical assessment of just how hassling each is to your life. For example:

If it's very important to you that you live in an area with good schools because you've got children, rate schools a 10 in terms of importance. Now rate the quality of your schools.

If your schools stack up to only about a 2, the difference between what you would like (a 10 times 10 situation) and what you've got (a 10 times 2 situation) is a great one (100 minus 20). It is this degree of discrepancy that Dr. Farmer's scoring system ingeniously takes into account. For indeed, the 65 degree to which any of us are bothered by our environment is directly proportional to the degree to which we care about it. Dr. Farmer's categories follow. (We'll walk you through the first category to get you started.)

Bureaucracies. If you don't mind gross incompetence on the part of the people responsible for instrumenting the legalities in your life, give the bureaucracies in your area a 5 or less in terms of their importance to you. But if administrative ineptitude drives you nuts, chalk up a 6 or above in the importance department.

Now decide just how bumbling the bureaucrats in your area really are. If you had to wait a month to get a permit just to put up a fence around your garden (and lost your lettuce in the interim), rate the buffoons responsible for that early harvest accordingly.

Have the idea? Two scores: one for importance, the other for quality. When you arrive at these ratings for each category, enter them on the score sheet.

The other hassle categories are as follows. (Kindly accept our exaggerated examples as representing "0" situations for quality.)

Shopping facilities. If securing a quart of milk requires the use of a gallon of gasoline, you're being hassled.

Crime. If an evening stroll in your neighborhood is looked upon as a form of suicide, you're being hassled.

Medical care. If a Doc Adams is all you've got (and he's hard to get sober), that's a hassle.

Commuting. If getting to work takes more out of you than being there, that qualifies as a hassle.

Repairmen. If the last time you called a plumber about a clogged toilet, he said, "Sure, bring it in," that, too, constitutes a hassle.

Neighbors. If you live next to a teenager who's practicing late into the night to become a rock star, there's a strong chance you're being hassled.

Utilities. If your telephone company staffs only one repairman (who also works another job), again, odds are you're being hassled.

Pollution. City living has its advantages, but black lung is not one of them. Daily "stay inside" air-quality ratings are definitely a hassle.

Recreation. If getting to the nearest opera would involve plane fare, you're being hassled.

Education. If school strikes have your 16-year-old still unsure of his multiplication tables, you (and he) are being hassled.

Climate. A three-bedroom Cape in Death Valley, for whatever price, is a hassle.

Those are Dr. Farmer's categories, which apply, for the most part, to living conditions. We must also work, however. And work, as we all know, can involve hassles. With Dr. Farmer's approval, we've added the following career-related considerations to his list of domestic ones.

Health. If, as much as you love being a vice president, you're not too happy about what it's doing to your body, you're being hassled. If your job is killing you, give it a 3 or less. But if it's giving you a kick in the rear to improve your health, give it a 7 or above.

Wealth. It's important to feel you're being paid what you think you're worth. If you're happy with your salary, give it a 7 or above. But if you're displeased with it, give it a 5 or less.

Happiness. It's what Dr. Farmer's Hassle Index is all about. A 10 if your life is immensely gratifying; a 0 if your spouse has to give you a pep talk to get you out of bed in the morning.

By having some fun with the Hassle Index, we have not meant to diminish its importance. Because what are hassles if not insidious forms of stress?

So what do we do about the hassles in our lives?

We do our best to eliminate or at least minimize them.

Is the Porsche really worth the time it spends in the shop? Might you not be happier in a more modest home closer to where you work?

These are, of course, questions that only you can answer—but you can't do that until you've at least asked them. Indeed, at the root of many of the hassles in our lives is the simple fact that we do not take the time to analyze them.

Why do you live and work as you do?

Must you live and work as you do?

They're tough questions, but life is too short not to answer them.

Your Hassle Index

To determine your overall Hassle Index (the higher the better), divide your total score by your highest possible score (determined by multiplying the sum total of your importance scores by 10).

For example: If your total score comes to 600, and the sum of your importance scores comes to 100, divide 600 by 100 times 10 (1,000). Your Hassle Index, in this case, would be 0.6. Got that?

$$\frac{\text{Total Score}}{\text{Highest Possible Score}} = \text{Your Hassle Index}$$

As we mentioned earlier, the closer your total score comes to equaling your highest possible score, the less hassle there is in your life. And so a score of 1.0 (100 percent) would be utopia. But Richard N. Farmer, Ph.D., creator of the Hassle Index, says that any score of 80 percent or above means you are living a life that is commendably hassle-free.

Hassle Index Score Sheet

Category	The Importance of It	The Quality of It	Combined Score (importance × quality)
Bureaucracies	_____	_____	_____
Shopping facilities	_____	_____	_____
Crime	_____	_____	_____
Medical care	_____	_____	_____
Commuting	_____	_____	_____
Repairmen	_____	_____	_____
Neighbors	_____	_____	_____
Utilities	_____	_____	_____
Pollution	_____	_____	_____
Recreation	_____	_____	_____
Education	_____	_____	_____
Climate	_____	_____	_____
Health	_____	_____	_____
Wealth	_____	_____	_____
Happiness	_____	_____	_____
		Total Score:	_____

PART II/
HOW TO KEEP
GOOD HABITS
FROM BORING YOU

Behind Good Health Is a Good Imagination

Our message so far has been that bad habits don't have to kill you, and that if you're willing to cultivate a little moderation, some can even be good for you. Because bad habits can provide pleasure, and pleasure is an essential nutrient to human life.

But good habits can provide pleasure, too—an even greater kind of pleasure, in fact, because good habits have the advantage of satisfying body and mind alike. When we comfort ourselves with bad habits, our bodies may say "delicious," but our minds are often having their doubts. When we learn to find pleasure in ways that we know are *good* for us, that element of doubt is removed.

Impossible, you say? There is simply no way that health foods can taste good? Or that exercise can be fun?

You're selling yourself short. "What the mind can conceive the body can achieve." I had a wrestling coach in high school who used to say that; and though it didn't make much of an impression on me at the time (perhaps because he would wait until the middle of some grueling conditioning routine to say it), it's become clear to me since that the man knew what he was talking about. Healthful foods are tasteless only if you allow them to be. And exercise is boring only if you lack the imagination to make it otherwise. Exercise never bothers me (anymore) because I've learned to think of it as a face-lift for my innards.

Superior health is a matter of putting our minds to work for the good of our bodies. And it's not as hard as it might sound because the same survival instinct that wants us happy *also* wants us healthy. As the Greek philosopher Epicurus said over two thousand years ago, "It is impossible to live pleasurably without also living wisely." Which means, simply, that it's hard to have a good time going out for ribs when your doctor has just told you to lose weight. As much as we've been programmed to pursue pleasure, we've *not* been geared to pursue it blindly—which is why the beer that takes the edge off a hangover on a Sunday afternoon never tastes as good as the one that celebrates a hard week's work on a Friday night. Our senses are dictated by our intellects more than we might sometimes care to admit.

Read through the following chapters with that in mind. Some of the good habits we'll be talking about may seem to take too much discipline, but give them time. And above all, give them thought. Knowing the nutritional advantages that an orange has over a doughnut really *can* make it taste sweeter; and knowing what's going on inside your body as you look absurd plodding around the block really can help you keep at it. Health has a very good friend in knowledge, but perhaps an even better one in imagination.

If there's a secret to living long, it's learning to find the pleasure you *want* from the food, exercise, and rest that you *need.*

SECTION I/FOOD

The key to a healthful diet is to eat foods that taste good and are good for us.

Impossible, you say?

We managed to do it throughout our evolution. And we can do it again now.

15/

How Healthful
Is the Way You Eat?

You may not be *exactly* what you eat, but you come pretty close. Good genes and a lust for life must also be considered, but even good genes and lust are at their best when well nourished.

With that in mind, we offer the following test. It should help you get some idea of how close to horrid your eating habits are, so that you may read the chapters that follow with some idea of the amount of work you have cut out for you. No cheating please.

1. On the average, I eat a serving of vegetables:
   A. less than once a day.
   B. at least once a day.
   C. twice a day.
   D. more than twice a day.
2. When at a restaurant, and the potatoes being offered are french fried, mashed, or baked, I normally choose:
   A. the french fried.
   B. the mashed.
   C. the baked.
3. The breakfast that most closely resembles my usual one is:
   A. a sweet roll and a cup of coffee.
   B. cold, presweetened cereal with milk, a glass of juice, and coffee.
   C. eggs and toast, a glass of juice, and coffee.
   D. a natural, whole grain cereal (such as oatmeal or granola) with milk, and a piece of fresh fruit.

4. Following my evening meal, I have a "junky" dessert (such as cake, pie, or ice cream):
   A. always.
   B. most of the time.
   C. some of the time.
   D. only on my birthday.

5. Most of the protein in my diet comes from·
   A. red meat.
   B. full-fat dairy products (such as whole milk and cheese).
   C. chicken and fish.
   D. a combination of chicken, fish, and/or a well-planned program of vegetable proteins (from beans, nuts, and grains).

6. The refined white sugar in my diet:
   A. comes from what I put in my coffee, on my cereal, the desserts I eat regularly, and the bonbons I munch on nightly.
   B. comes from what is hidden in the processed foods I eat.
   C. is minimal; I make a strong effort to get very little refined white sugar in my diet.

7. If I'm hungry, and there's nothing but a vending machine around:
   A. I'll have a candy bar.
   B. I'll have a pack of crackers.
   C. I'll have a bag of peanuts.
   D. I won't have anything at all.

8. The last time I had something like a Twinkie was:
   A. I am having something like a Twinkie right now
   B. when I was living on $5 a week in college.
   C. when I was in grade school.
   D. I do not even know what a Twinkie is.

9. I eat potato chips and/or pretzels:
   A. regularly.
   B. only at parties.
   C. never.

10. I consider fried and/or greasy foods:
    A. a delicious part of my regular diet.
    B. okay to enjoy occasionally.
    C. something to avoid like the plague.

How to Score

Give yourself 1 point for every A answer; 2 points for every B, 3 for each C, and 4 for any D. Now add up your points.

A score of 36 is perfect. You may have a hot fudge sundae (if you can keep it down). Congratulations.

A score of 10 is abominable. It means you are violating every nutritional rule in the book.

As for all of you who fall somewhere in between, you may think of yourselves as follows:

35–30 Honorably health conscious.
29–25 Commendably health conscious.
24–20 Acceptably health conscious.
19–15 Health *un*conscious.
14–10 Reprehensibly health *un*conscious.

16/
An Un-Diet

If your score on the preceding test has you thinking some major changes are in order, do not make the mistake of biting off more than you can chew. If you want to improve your diet—permanently—you're best off keeping as many of your current eating habits as possible, particularly if you're trying to lose weight.

"People who go on fad or crash diets do themselves a disservice in more ways than one," says Covert Bailey, author of *Fit or Fat?* (Houghton Mifflin, 1978). "When someone fasts or adheres to an unbalanced diet, he puts his body in a kind of emergency state which can actually make whatever food he does eat more fattening." The process, Bailey says, is a holdover from our caveman days when the only time we ate poorly was when we *had* to, in times of famine.

"The body hasn't forgotten those times yet," Bailey claims. "It still associates inadequate food intake with famine—time to slow the metabolism down and *store* rather than use."

So do not make the error of signaling "famine" to your body by rushing headlong into a jungle of salad greens. Your eating patterns have been a lifetime in the making, so they are not going to be overnight in the breaking.

Do you enjoy a bowl of ice cream before bed?

Fine. Try filling that bowl with yogurt next time, though, instead of maple walnut.

Do you enjoy a couple of drinks after work?

How hard would it be to make "one" your new definition of a couple?

Get the idea? Minor changes rather than major monkey wrenches. A pound of fat yields 3,500 calories, which means that by reducing your calorie intake by as little as 200 a day, you can be 20 pounds thinner in a year.

Not fast enough for you?

Careful. The danger in losing weight much faster than that is that you don't prepare yourself for the day you reach your desired goal. What then? Is it going to be liquid protein forever?

It is not uncommon for people to lose and regain as much as 1,000 pounds seesawing their way through fad diets. And that's bad because weight loss on diets that do not involve exercise usually involves considerable *muscle* loss. When weight is regained, though, it's usually in the form of pure fat. The 75 seesaw ride, in other words, makes you wind up *fatter* for all your efforts.

"But can't I just lose a quick ten pounds, then go back to my normal way of eating, without gaining it back?"

We wish we could say yes, but a higher authority—your body—says no. Because by losing those ten pounds, you become a smaller person. And the smaller you are, the fewer calories you need. It's only a matter of time before your old way of eating will have you back to your old way of weighing.

To lose weight, or just to improve your diet in general, you're going to have to make changes you can live with. And to do that, you're going to have to achieve a compromise between two undeniable aspects of your soul: the you that wants a healthful diet and the you that wants a satisfying one. There can be no inner peace, and hence no permanent improvements, until that treaty is made.

And how can it be done?

Subtly, as we've said. If weight loss is your primary concern, rest assured that it's becoming increasingly clear to doctors and patients alike that the longer weight loss takes, the longer it lasts. The track records of most quick weight loss programs are so dismal, in fact, that we feel totally confident in offering you a nearly opposite alternative; an "un-diet," a collection of very general guidelines by which you improve your diet at your own pace—and to the degree that you decide is right for you. It merely involves making minor substitutions, learning to eat *better* if not necessarily less. After all, if you're unhappy with your current relationship with food, it's probably for the potentially healthful reason that you simply like to eat. Master the un-diet and you can get that urge working *for* rather than against you, because the un-diet is as healthful as it is slimming. Enough philosophy. Here are the guiding principles of the un-diet.

- *Make up your mind, first of all, that you really want to make some dietary changes.* Because if you don't, you won't—no matter how easy we make things for you.
- *Begin your un-diet at the supermarket.* You can't eat what you don't have.
- *Make a list of priorities.* Decide which foods you love most, and eat them with respect. The foods to cut out are the ones you may be taking for granted: i.e., the sour cream on your potato that *for 17 calories less* could be yogurt; the butter on your broccoli that *for 102 calories* could be lemon juice.
- *Learn to harbor ill thoughts about sugar.* It's a weight-loser's worst enemy. In addition to being virtually devoid of nutrients, its calories (about 15 per teaspoon) can arouse feelings of false hunger by causing the pancreas to release inordinate amounts of insulin.

- *Realize that sugar can travel in strange company* and by other names: corn syrup, invert sugar, dextrose, and maltose. They're all basically the same thing, and they're in many more processed foods (crackers, frozen pizza, canned soups) than you may realize.
- *Exercise.* You don't have to, but you're dumb not to, because not only does exercise burn calories, it tones and strengthens muscles. And people who have a higher percentage of muscle than fat burn up more calories *even when they're resting.* (See box on page 78.)
- *Learn how many calories there are* in four ounces of fish, then forget it. You're out to make healthful eating a habit, remember, not a career. Familiarize yourself with enough food facts to know your friends from your enemies, then get down to the more serious business of enjoying.
- *Eat more water.* It's our only food that has no calories at all, and it's most abundant in vegetables and fruit. (A carrot stick is about 90 percent water whereas a pretzel is about five.)
- *Drink less alcohol.* Notice we did not say *no* alcohol. That might be asking too much. What we *do* ask, though, is that you at least be conscious of pure alcohol as the ultimate junk food— nutritionally destitute but calorically loaded.
- *Start thinking of food as something that becomes part of you.* Logic like this can be helpful in depriving bonbons of some of their charm.
- *Chew a lot;* it's less fattening than swallowing. Chewing takes time, as does digestion, so by thoroughly chewing *whatever* it is you eat, you give your stomach more time to let you know it's getting full.
- *Look to fiber* (more often than Turkish taffy) to help you do this chewing. In addition to filling you up, the fiber in bulky foods such as whole grain products, vegetables, and fruits can actually make other foods you eat less fattening by affecting the way dietary fats get digested.
- *Put a premium on foods that are natural.* And by that we mean foods that haven't been run through the mill by technology. Potato chips, for example, have 6 times as many calories, 250 times as much salt, and 400 times as much fat as potatoes eaten baked. And they also cost about 10 times as much.
- *Start counting condiments.* There are more calories in the amount of dressing that most people put on their salads than there are in their salads. Mayonnaise, vegetable oils, butter, margarine— they've all got about 100 calories a tablespoon. Simply by not buttering your two pieces of toast in the morning, you could be

ten pounds thinner this same time next year. (See box on page 80.)

- *Make a connection between the "fat" in food and "fat" on people.* The former contributes heavily to the latter, because at nine calories per gram, fat is more than twice as fattening as carbohydrates or protein.
- *Allow yourself splurges.* Call them rewards, though. There must be room in *any* dietary program for *guilt-free* celebration.
- *Don't eat if you're not hungry.* Three meals a day is a relatively recent and arbitrary convention. If you're not hungry when a mealtime rolls around, don't eat. You're better off listening to your body than you are to someone in the kitchen.
- *Try not to eat alone.* Eating with other people tends to slow you down, and it also puts you in a position of "accountability" for your imbibings.

Exercise: Maybe the Best Diet Food of All

Which of the following do you think would be a better way of losing weight: eating less or exercising more?

If you said eating less, that could be why you're still overweight. Exercise is the better approach because it helps fix what makes us fat in the first place: our metabolisms.

Muscle tissue consumes more calories than any other type of tissue in the body. During moments of extreme exertion, its energy requirements can leap fifty fold. Fat tissue, by comparison, lays relatively dormant. "Clearly, if you want to get rid of calories, you should look to the quantity and quality of your muscle."

Those words come from Covert Bailey, author of *Fit or Fat?* (Houghton Mifflin, 1978), who has looked at weight gain from the inside out. Most people get fat, he says, because they have allowed their muscles to get lazy when it comes to consuming calories. Regular daily exercise— even if it's as little as 12 minutes' worth a day, he says—keeps enzymes inside muscle tissue alert to making use of passing sources of energy in the bloodstream.

In an unconditioned person, Bailey explains, muscle tissue loses its appetite. Biochemically speaking, that happens as unconditioned muscle cells become less sensitive to insulin, a substance whose job it is to stimulate body cells to open the pores in muscle tissue for the entrance of blood sugar. And fewer open pores in muscle cells mean more sugar wandering about in the bloodstream to be picked up by . . .

You guessed it, fat cells. "With the muscle cells rejecting the glucose, the fat tissue becomes a glucose sink," Bailey says. And once inside fat

- *Think before you eat.* Few of us do. To avoid the "I wish I hadn'ts," try a few more "maybe I shouldn'ts."
- *Have a heart-to-heart talk with your taste buds.* Tell them how much better for you an apple is than a cupcake. We think you'll be surprised at how willing they are to listen.
- *Don't be afraid to eat out.* There's no reason that, with some polite instruction, you can't have it "your way" wherever you go.
- *Respect your inalienable right to feel satisfied.* There is nothing wrong with feeling good after you've eaten. There *is* something wrong, however, with not giving your body a chance to get this good feeling from foods that also happen to be good for you.

If all this sounds too easy, that's why it can work. Most diets fail because they're too hard. And you work hard enough as it is.

---

cells, glucose becomes instrumental in the conversion of glycerol and fatty acids to triglyceride, which is the neutral, stable kind of fat that the body is composed of.

Exercise, moreover, makes muscle cells better at using the glucose they do get by encouraging the growth of calorie-consuming enzymes. "People who are getting in shape with regular exercise are increasing these enzymes, whereas people who are getting more out of shape day by day, are slowly losing theirs because they aren't needed," Bailey says.

(In light of this, Bailey—an avid runner—will sometimes offer biochemical encouragement to himself on the road: "Grow you enzymes, grow.")

To fix what's making us fat in the first place, then, we need *moderate* daily exercise. We emphasize the word moderate because in an unconditioned person just starting out, vigorous exercise will not encourage the kind of biochemical activity necessary to burn fat most effectively. When made to exercise strenuously, a fat person's metabolism will reach for blood sugar, rather than blood fats, for energy. So walking is the ideal fat-burning exercise for overweight and out-of-condition people. "If I were grossly fat, I would give up whatever was necessary—job, housework, whatever—and walk three to four hours per day," Bailey says.

Enzymes, then, are the key to fighting fat. And to get them, we need to exercise. But we *also* need to eat. Many crash diets defeat themselves, Bailey says, by not supplying us with the nutrients we need for adequate enzyme growth.

Good food *and* good exercise: It may not be the only way, but it's the best way. Losing fat is more active a process than most diets give us the energy for.

Condiments: Caloric Clowns

Condiments can fool you, because you use them without thinking. And worse yet, without remembering. "Only had a piece of toast for breakfast," you congratulate yourself as you wait hungrily in the cafeteria line for lunch . . .

Like fun. You had a piece of toast and its caloric equivalent all over again in butter. That's the absurdity of condiments. Some have as many —if not *more*—calories than the foods we put them on.

Take a look at these condiments and their calories. What we've tried to do is put the spotlight on those "non-foods" that (calorie-wise) could be making up a considerably larger portion of your food intake than you realize. Many, in addition to being high in calories, are also high in fat —those at the top especially. Oils, butter, margarine, mayonnaise, and tartar sauce (for anyone concerned about being overweight) should be avoided at all cost.

As for the others, the best approach might be simply to ask yourself: "Is the amount of taste I'm getting really worth the calories?"

Probably not. Which is what really makes condiments ridiculous. Do yourself a favor and find out how good food can be without them.

Condiments and Their Caloric Content

	Calories*
Vegetable oil	120
Butter	102
Margarine	101
Mayonnaise	99
Tartar sauce	74
Honey	64
Jams and preserves	54
Cream cheese	52
Sugar	51
Maple syrup	50
Cream, light	29
Pickle relish, sweet	21
Steak sauce	21
Ketchup	16
Mustard, brown	15
Barbecue sauce	12
Worcestershire sauce	12

NOTE: *Per tablespoon of condiment cited.

SOURCES: Adapted from U.S. Department of Agriculture Handbook nos. 8-1, 8-4, 8-6, and 456; and USDA Nutrient Data Research Group, 1981.

17/

A Crash Course in Carbohydrates

No, you do not yet understand carbohydrates. Because if you did, you would know:

- whether or not they're fattening;
- how they can be in foods as dissimilar as candy bars, grapefruit, milk, lima beans, doughnuts, celery, and whole wheat bread;
- what the differences are between simple carbohydrates, complex carbohydrates, refined carbohydrates, unrefined carbohydrates, sugar, starch, fructose, fiber, the starch in your muscles, the sugar in milk, the sugar in beer, and the sugar in your blood.

Getting a feel, now, for your ignorance?

Good, because maybe now we can get you straightened out. And it's important that we do because what you *think* you know about carbohydrates could hurt you. Indeed, some advertisers would have us believe that chocolate bars and white bread are as healthfully energizing as fresh fruit and brown rice. It's just not so.

Depending on *how* you get your carbohydrates, in fact, you could wind up anywhere from lean and healthy to fat and malnourished. Some doctors go as far as to say that eating the wrong kinds of carbohydrate foods sets you up for any number of diseases—heart disease, cancer of the colon, and diabetes, to name just a few. But more on that later.

First we'd like to explain what carbohydrates are and how they function. Because not until you understand *that* can you intelligently decide which ones to avoid.

Carbohydrates, first of all, are not foods; they are molecular compounds *in* foods. A potato, for example, gets called a carbohydrate, but there is also protein and a little bit of fat in a potato. Breads, crackers, chocolate bars, ice cream, cereals, pastry, and fruit are the same way. They are not carbohydrates, but rather foods *rich* in carbohydrates. The only foods that are pure carbohydrate, in fact, are table sugar, honey, some jellies and jams, some candies and syrups.

Now we start splitting hairs. . . .

Carbohydrates do not come in just one form: They come in at least 16. The only reason they all get called carbohydrates is that they all consist of varying combinations of carbon, hydrogen, and oxygen atoms. Leave it to nature, though, to arrange those three atoms in some miraculously dissimilar ways. The cellulose that goes "crunch" in celery, for example, is a carbohydrate. But then so is the maple syrup you pour all over your pancakes.

Nutritionists have been able to squeeze these 16 major nutritional carbohydrates into two basic categories: simple and complex. The simple carbohydrates are the kind in sugar, fruit, milk, and, to some degree, vegetables. They taste sweet, and the reason they're called simple is because—molecularly speaking—that's what they are. Which is why they digest so quickly. There are not many chemical bonds to be broken before simple carbohydrates can be absorbed by the bloodstream, and so they burn quickly.

Complex carbohydrates, on the other hand, are more . . . complex. They are made up of *hundreds* of molecules of simple carbohydrates linked together, and so they take longer to digest. Which is why a baked potato's 100 calories stick with you longer than the 120 or so in a candy bar; they take longer for your body to break down into a usable form. Complex carbohydrates are most prevalent in breads, cereals, beans, root vegetables (such as potatoes and carrots), pasta, and rice—foods we commonly call starches.

Now for the sorrowful tale of refinement.

If nutrients could sue for damages, carbohydrates would be millionaires. There was a time when there was no such thing as a carbohydrate food that was unhealthful. Not until modern-day food processors came along and started taking the protein, vitamins, minerals, and fiber *out* of carbohydrate foods was it possible to get your hands on one that was bad for you. Reach for a carbohydrate food now, though, and it's apt to be regrettably incomplete: plenty of calories, but sadly lacking in the nutrients necessary to put those calories to good use.

Why are carbohydrate foods refined?

In the case of flour made from grains, it's to make it better for baking. Baked goods made from refined flour are lighter and fluffier. And refined flours, because their natural oils have been removed, can be stored without turning rancid.

In the case of sugar, refinement is simply the most expedient way of getting sugar cane and sugar beets into a form that can be used as an additive. The average American now consumes over 90 pounds of refined sugar a year —two-thirds of which comes by way of processed foods.

The food industry does make efforts to restore some of the nutrients that refinement strips, however—a procedure called "enrichment" or "fortification." One nutrient that it doesn't restore, though, is fiber. And fiber is what carbohydrate foods are all about. They are, in fact, our *sole source* of this all-important material. Without it, we're in trouble.

"The normal human diet has always been high in fiber, and our digestive systems evolved to rely on this common part of food, even though it only passes through our bodies and emerges in a form quite similar to that which it entered," says Sanford Siegal, D.O., M.D., author of *Dr. Siegal's Natural Fiber Permanent Weight-Loss Diet* (Dial Press/James Wade, 1975). Indeed, it's been estimated that our prehistoric ancestors consumed about 25 grams of dietary fiber a day. In our modern-day world we're lucky if we get one-fifth that much.

The results of this fiber shortage? Not good. Because it leads to:

- increased rates of coronary artery disease—because fiber has been shown to keep cholesterol out of the blood by inhibiting its absorption in the intestine.
- increased rates of cancer of the colon. Fiber's protective effect here is to speed potential carcinogens through the large intestine, thus reducing the chance of their causing damage.
- obesity. Fiber is a carbohydrate that has no calories, because it doesn't get digested. What's more, it has the ability to take even some of the *other* calories *out* of the foods we eat by inhibiting the absorption of dietary fats.
- diverticular disease. By keeping us regular, fiber can prevent us from "straining at stool," an unpleasantry that can cause ruptures of the walls of the large intestine (a serious problem for one-third of Americans over the age of 45).
- diabetes. Diets high in rapidly digested fiberless sugars may in time impair the workings of the pancreas, whose job it is to produce enough insulin to see that these sugars get properly utilized.

Fiber, in short, is a very crucial nutrient. And refined carbohydrates just don't have enough of it.

So what does it all mean?

It means fruit instead of candy. Whole wheat bread instead of white. More beans, brown rice, high-fiber cereals, and real potatoes. Fewer doughnuts, lily-white dinner rolls, lighter-than-air pancakes, and instant potatoes.

Carbohydrate foods don't *have* to be unhealthful. They have the potential, in fact, of being among the most healthful foods we can eat—low in fat and calories and high in vitamins, minerals, and fiber. Indeed, if there's been a nutrient misunderstood by the American public, it's been the carbohydrate. It's time the record got set straight.

But Are They Fattening?

Carbohydrates—regardless of whether they're simple or complex, refined or unrefined—contain four calories per gram, which is the same as protein and about five calories *less* per gram than fat. So how did carbohydrates get the reputation for being fattening?

Because about ten years ago, a certain "Drinking Man's Diet" came along and said, "Here, have all the fatty meats, cheese, mayonnaise, butter, and booze you want—but avoid carbohydrates—and you'll lose weight."

This deal, as it turns out, proved to be a little like the one offered by the Devil. People lost weight—but they also lost health. Kidney disorders, loss of muscle tissue, fatigue, and dizziness were among some of the less talked about items on these low-carbohydrate, high-fat menus.

The damage to foods containing carbohydrates, however, had been done. Beans got blacklisted along with bonbons. Potatoes got pushed aside like pastry. Carbohydrates—in *any* form—had been "framed" as the ringleaders of obesity.

What the Drinking Man's Diet had failed to consider was that not all types of carbohydrates get digested in the same way, and so not all types contribute equally to weight gain.

Simple carbohydrate foods, particularly refined ones, get digested so fast that they are very *unfilling*. (We'll include table sugar, jellies, candy, and highly sugared pastries in that category.) Even complex carbohydrate foods (starches) that have been refined can get pretty "slippery." (White bread, for example, spends less time in the stomach than whole wheat.) So . . .

In terms of how quickly *refined* carbohydrate foods get digested, yes, they too can be fattening. You would, for example, be better off satisfying an afternoon hunger pang with 200 calories (about two ounces) of cheese than you would with 200 calories of candy—reason being that the fat and protein in cheese take considerably longer to digest than the refined simple carbohydrates (mainly sucrose) in candy.

How does fructose (fruit sugar) fit into the carbohydrate picture?

It's a simple carbohydrate (like table sugar), but it gets absorbed more slowly than table sugar. It's also less likely to contribute to the formation of plaque involved in the development of cavities. So even though a large apple may contain more total sugar than a candy bar, that sugar—mainly in the form of fructose—is more healthful. Then, too, the apple is loaded with fiber. The candy bar (unless it's got peanuts) has none.

Don't Stop Eating Carbohydrate Foods—Simply Have . . .

These	Portion	Carbo-hydrates (grams)	Crude fiber* (grams)	Calories
Brown rice	1 cup	49.7	0.6	232
Potato, baked	1 medium	32.8	1.2	145
Whole wheat bread	2 slices	23.8	0.8	122
Oatmeal	1 cup	23.3	0.5	132
Bran muffin	1	17.2	0.7	104
Apple	1 medium	30.7	2.3	123
Carrot	1	7.0	0.8	30
Whole wheat pancake	4" diameter	9.2	0.2	62
Popcorn	1 cup	5.3	0.2	41
Peanuts	10	3.7	0.7	105

Instead of These	Portion	Carbo-hydrates (grams)	Crude fiber* (grams)	Calories
White rice	1 cup	49.6	0.2	223
French fries	10	28.1	0.8	214
White bread	2 slices	27.2	0.1	148
Corn flakes, sugarcoated	1 cup	36.5	0.2	154
Doughnut, cake type	1 plain	29.8	trace	227
Candy bar, fudge/caramel/peanuts	1 ounce	18.2	0.1	123
Saltine crackers	4	8.0	trace	48
Waffle, frozen	4" diameter	9.2	trace	56
Pretzels	10	22.8	0.1	117
Potato chips	10	10.0	0.3	114

NOTE: *Crude fiber is cellulose.

SOURCES: Adapted from U.S. Department of Agriculture Handbook nos. 8 and 456.

18/

In Defense of Vitamins

Not since Darwin, perhaps, has a scientific issue ruffled the medical community the way vitamins have. Do we need to take them or not?

Traditionalists say no—we can get all the nutrients we need from the foods we eat.

A growing number of dissenters, however, disagree. Vitamin supplements, they say, are necessary because our bodies are being stressed by environmental pollutants and because processing is taking out of our foods the nutrients that our tired soils are having trouble putting in.

Who's right?

That depends on who's defining the word "need."

If it's the federal government, and our needs are, as they say, adequately represented by the latest set of RDAs, then yes, you could—if you were careful—get all the vitamins and minerals the government says are "adequate to meet the known nutritional needs of practically all healthy persons." But if you would like your health to be *more* than just adequate . . . or if you have some bad habits—or bad genes—that distinguish you from "practically all healthy persons," then the government's RDAs may *not* be enough. And that is what the great vitamin debate is all about.

"The RDAs were originally designed to insure that large segments of the population would not develop serious nutritional deficiencies," notes Alan R. Gaby, M.D., a physician from Kent, Washington. They are "minimum requirements for minimal health," and in no way do they attempt to answer the question of whether larger amounts can bestow larger benefits, Dr. Gaby says.

Which, of course, is precisely what a growing number of researchers believe nutritional supplements can do. Those experimenters have not had a lot of support from the scientific community, but they have persisted nonetheless, encouraged by their findings. We quote from a letter written by one such revolutionary, an M.D., to the *Medical Tribune* (February 7, 1979):

Like most physicians I believed that most people got the vitamins they needed from their food. Then I started to read Pauling, Williams, Irwin Stone, and Carlton Fredericks. I started giving vitamin supplements to my patients with various forms of joint pains, peripheral vascular disease, angina pectoris—with very good results with most of them. One patient with unstable angina, whom I was ready to send to the surgeons for a bypass, improved so much on multivitamins—vitamin C, vitamin E, and lecithin—that he can now run around the block a few times without experiencing angina.

I told my colleagues . . . and most of them started thinking of me as a quack. I realize that they feel this way because they follow the lead of the AMA [American Medical Association], the FDA [Federal Drug Administration], and the respected leaders in the medical profession. The general attitude is: If the medical establishment doesn't know it, then it's either wrong or not worth knowing. This attitude, I feel, is one of the reasons why, after many years and billions of dollars' worth of research, we haven't made any significant dent in the treatment and prevention—especially prevention—of cancer and other degenerative diseases, such as cardiovascular disease and arthritis.

The AMA counter to that sort of testimony has been that there is an enormous placebo effect at play, that controlled clinical and laboratory studies to support such evidence do not exist, and that such evidence for the most part comes from sources outside the scientific community.

Such objections, however, have not daunted vitamin takers. "The American public is way ahead of the doctors on this one," says John Francis Catchpool, a "renegade" M.D. from Sausalito, California.

Why should the medical community be resistant to such a promising new field?

There are several theories.

Some critics say it's a simple case of monetary greed. "It's more profitable to fix things that are broken than to keep them running smoothly in the first place," the argument goes. Hence the medical world's greater expertise at taking apart hearts than putting together meals.

To others, however, that assessment seems a bit harsh. David Rubin, M.D., a professor of preventive medicine at Georgetown University, sees the medical profession's current disinterest in nutrition as the result of a system of education that's hospital-oriented, a system "where there are acute problems, and you teach students how to care for people who are already sick" (*Caveat Emptor*, July, 1980).

Jonathan Wright, M.D. (with whom we discussed the issue by phone), agreed: "Doctors today are trained to look for singular cures for singular problems. And nutritional therapy just doesn't always work that way. It may correct a specific condition, but it does so by benefiting the entire organism.

"Most M.D.'s see vitamins as being of value only in cases of gross deficiencies. But there are many specific instances of defective enzymes or metabolic abnormalities where more would be beneficial. It's our belief that vitamins and minerals are enzyme inducers and hormone modulators, which means they can promote beneficial metabolic processes with varying amounts given."

When we asked Dr. Wright how he became interested in nutritional therapy, he said, "By studying on my own, *after* medical school." And when we asked him why he decided to employ nutritional therapy in his practice, he said, "Because it worked."

Dr. Gaby, an associate of Dr. Wright's, suspects that it could be this very fact—that vitamins *do* work—that has the medical profession reluctant to promote them. Vitamins, by giving patients power to treat themselves, may represent a threat to the medical profession's degree of control.

Indeed, the medical community has not been the least bit coy about the back seat it has given nutrition in its educational program.

"Most medical schools devote less than three hours of total instruction to nutritional deficiency and therapy," admitted Richard A. Wright, M.D., in an editorial in the *Journal of the American Medical Association* (August 8, 1980). "The area of nutrition has been neglected by the medical profession."

Following testimony given at a Senate subcommittee meeting on the subject of nutrition being taught in medical schools, Senator Patrick J. Leahy of Vermont is reported to have remarked, "There was far, far more time in the average medical school spent on the question of malpractice insurance . . . than there was on nutrition" (*Caveat Emptor,* July, 1980).

That's a little scary. Particularly in light of current estimates that six out of the ten leading causes of death in this country are diet-related.

Does the medical profession have any plans for wising up?

Not in the immediate future, it doesn't. Many medical school administrators, unfortunately, still regard nutrition as a passing fad. Others are using the excuse that medical school curricula are simply too full to allow for additional fields of study.

"In order to get nutrition education in medical schools," one government official has said, "enlightened students and faculty are going to have to conduct a guerrilla effort."

In the meantime, don't be surprised if your doctor gives you the impression he thinks vitamins are a joke. He simply hasn't had the training to think otherwise. It's going to be up to *you* to pay attention to your diet—and supplement it in areas you suspect might be weak.

What Are Vitamins, Anyway?

Vitamins are microscopic compounds that serve as essential links in the trillions of chemical reactions that go on inside our bodies every second. Without them, those chemical reactions either happen improperly—or they don't happen at all. For example, a molecule of glucose (blood sugar) could bump into a molecule of the enzyme that breaks down glucose in your body. But unless a molecule of vitamin B_6 (thiamine) were around to spice that meeting up, it would go very poorly. And so, ultimately, would you.

Dr. Williams's Recommended Vitamin Supplementation

	RDA for Men*	RDA for Women*	Suggested Supplementation for Adults
Vitamin A (I.U.)	3,330	2,664	7,500
Thiamine (milligrams)	1.4	1.0	2.0
Riboflavin (milligrams)	1.6	1.2	2.0
Niacin (milligrams)	18	13	20
Vitamin B_6 (milligrams)	2.2	2.0	3.0
Vitamin B_{12} (micrograms)	3.0	3.0	9.0
Vitamin C (milligrams)	60	60	250
Vitamin D (I.U.)	200	200	400
Vitamin E (I.U.)	15	12	40

NOTES: *Ages 23 to 50.
I.U.—international units.
RDA—Recommended Dietary Allowances.

SOURCES: Adapted from *Physicians' Handbook of Nutritional Science,* by Roger J. Williams (Springfield, Ill.: Charles C. Thomas, 1975); and *Recommended Dietary Allowances,* 9th ed. (Washington, D.C.: National Academy of Sciences, 1980).

The other B vitamins behave in the same way—as catalysts, meaning they improve the speed and efficiency of key molecular interactions, many of which have to do with the release of energy from carbohydrates.

Not all the vitamins, however, are only matchmakers. Vitamins A and E, for example, also act as chaperones, making sure that the body's molecular social life doesn't get out of hand. Chemists call these vitamins antioxidants, which means they keep oxygen molecules from getting involved in chemical reactions they shouldn't.

Then there's paternal vitamin D, which oversees the body's absorption of calcium. And the very busy vitamin C, whose duties include fighting infection and strengthening connective tissue.

Vitamins, in short, are elements in food that make food work. Without them, proteins, fats, and carbohydrates wouldn't know what to do with themselves. British sailors back in the sixteenth century died on 4,000 calories a day of biscuits, salted meat, dried fish, cheese, butter, and beer—a graphic demonstration of the fact that man lives not by calories alone. Because those men were deficient in vitamin C, they died of scurvy. But they might as well have starved to death.

Indeed, human nutrition is a more complex and demanding affair than many of us might care to think. It is *not* merely a matter of getting a good balance of macronutrients (proteins, carbohydrates, and fats). It necessitates including a proper balance of micronutrients (vitamins and minerals) to put those macronutrients to work.

And what's the best way to do that?

By getting a good mix of all types of food—fruits, vegetables, dairy products, whole grains, and lean meats—and then paying close attention to your body to see if that's enough. If you're uncommonly robust, it might be. But —if you are less than flawless at absorbing vitamins (which many of us are); or if you smoke (which robs the body of vitamin C); or drink large amounts of coffee or alcohol (both are hard on B vitamins); or live in a polluted environment (which could call for additional A, C, and E); or are under a lot of stress (a glutton for B vitamins and C); or are taking birth control pills (also tough on some B vitamins)—then supplementation might be a good idea.

How much?

Again, that depends on you and your lifestyle. Roger J. Williams, Ph.D., D.Sc., one of the world's leading experts in vitamin research, has proposed what he feels would be reasonably safe coverage for most reasonably healthy people. It is, as you can see in the preceding table, more copious than the Recommended Dietary Allowances—particularly in light of the fact that Dr. Williams suggests these levels to be taken in *addition* to what you get if you eat a typical American diet.

19/

The Whole Story on Fiber

In 20 words or less, define fiber.

If you said, "the indigestible part of food that makes it easier to have a bowel movement," give yourself a score of 50 percent and pay attention. There is more to the fiber story than you're being told on your box of bran cereal.

As the Institute of Food Technologists' Panel on Food Safety and Nutrition puts it, "There are such great differences in the physiological effects of the various constituents of dietary fiber that it is almost meaningless to discuss the benefits of a high-fiber diet [without making distinctions between them]."

What this means is: Not all fiber works with the brute force of wheat bran, or the obvious indigestibility of corn on the cob. The kind that does, as a matter of fact, is in the minority. Most fiber works on a level much more microscopic than the word "roughage" implies.

Which is why half a cup of cooked spinach can have as much fiber as a bowl of shredded wheat. And why one medium banana can provide more roughage than four cups of popcorn. Fiber can be very tiny stuff. Tiny enough to be unaffected by chewing. Aside from a few exceptions (corn being one), the fiber story is best told on a molecular scale.

Dietary vs. Crude Fiber

What's the difference? Like night and day.

- Crude fiber is what's left over when a food is digested artificially in the lab. Dietary fiber is what's left over when a food is digested—for real—in the human gut.
- Crude fiber includes only the most rugged—cellulose and lignin. Dietary fiber encompasses all types, including the more fragile hemicelluloses, gums, pectic substances and mucilages, and other types of carbohydrates.
- Crude fiber is chemically inert. Most of the dietary fibers are chemically active.

91

(continued on page 94)

Fiber Content of Selected Foods

	Portion	Dietary Fiber (grams)	Calories
Cereal, 100 percent bran	1 cup	19.9	132
Apricots, dried	½ cup	15.6	169
Prunes, dried	5	8.2	130
Apple	1 medium	7.9	80
Broccoli, cooked	1 medium stalk	7.4	47
Coconut	2″ × 2″ piece	6.1	156
Spinach, cooked	½ cup	5.7	21
Blackberries	½ cup	5.3	42
Almonds	¼ cup	5.1	212
Pinto beans, raw	¼ cup	4.8	166
Red raspberries	½ cup	4.6	35
Shredded wheat	1 cup	4.3	124
Peas, cooked	½ cup	4.2	57
Banana	1 medium	4.0	101
Dates, dried	¼ cup	3.9	122
Potato, baked	1 medium	3.9	145
Pear	1 medium	3.8	100
Lentils, cooked	½ cup	3.7	106
Corn, cooked	1 ear	3.6	70
Lima beans, cooked	½ cup	3.5	126
Sweet potato, cooked	1 medium	3.5	172
Apple pie	⅛	3.1	302
Blackberry pie	⅛	3.1	287
Peanuts	¼ cup	2.9	210
Brown rice, raw	¼ cup	2.8	180
Corn flakes	1 cup	2.8	97
Oats, rolled	½ cup	2.8	156
Orange	1 medium	2.6	64
Raisins	¼ cup	2.5	105
Brussels sprouts, cooked	4	2.4	30
Navy beans, raw	¼ cup	2.4	174
Peanut butter	2 tablespoons	2.4	188
Whole wheat bread	1 slice	2.4	61
Apricots, fresh	3 medium	2.3	55
Carrot, raw	1 medium	2.3	30
Beets, cooked	½ cup	2.1	27
Peach	1 medium	2.1	58
Kale greens, cooked	½ cup	2.0	22
Summer squash, raw	½ cup	2.0	13
Zucchini, raw	½ cup	2.0	11
Parsnips, cooked	½ cup	1.9	51
Snap beans, raw	½ cup	1.9	18
Tomato, raw	1 medium	1.8	27

	Portion	Dietary Fiber (grams)	Calories
Turnips, cooked	½ cup	1.7	18
Barley, raw	⅛ cup	1.6	87
Okra, raw	½ cup	1.6	18
Strawberries	½ cup	1.6	28
Tangerine	1 medium	1.6	39
Walnuts	¼ cup	1.6	196
Chili con carne, canned, prepared with water	1 cup	1.5	169
Green pepper, raw	1 large	1.5	36
Black bean soup, canned, prepared with water	1 cup	1.3	116
Fruit salad, canned	½ cup	1.3	43
Wheat bran	1 tablespoon	1.3	6
Cherries, sweet	10	1.1	47
Endive	1 cup	1.1	10
Cauliflower, raw	½ cup	1.0	14
Pineapple	¾" slice	1.0	44
White rice, raw	¼ cup	1.0	177
Asparagus, cooked	4 medium	0.9	12
Cabbage, raw	½ cup	0.9	9
Mushrooms, raw	½ cup	0.9	10
Popcorn, popped	1 cup	0.9	23
Sprouts	¼ cup	0.8	12
White bread	1 slice	0.8	76
Big Mac	1	0.7	541
Celery, raw	1 stalk	0.7	7
Cream of asparagus soup, canned, prepared with water	1 cup	0.7	87
Pea soup, canned, prepared with water	1 cup	0.7	164
Grapefruit	½ medium	0.6	40
Onions, raw	¼ cup	0.6	16
Plum	3 medium	0.6	20
Grapes, seedless	10	0.5	34
Minestrone soup, canned, prepared with water	1 cup	0.4	79
Cucumber	½ cup	0.2	8
Cayenne	⅛ teaspoon	0.1	0.8
Chili powder	⅛ teaspoon	0.1	1

SOURCES: Adapted from *McCance and Widdowson's The Composition of Foods*, by A. A. Paul and D. A. T. Southgate (New York: Elsevier/North-Holland Biomedical Press, 1978); "Composition of Foods Commonly Used in Diets for Persons with Diabetes," by James W. Anderson, Wen-Ju Lin, and Kyleen Ward (*Diabetes Care*, September/October, 1978); and U.S. Department of Agriculture Handbook nos. 8-2, 8-6, and 456.

- Crude fiber moves through you with the subtlety of a bulldozer. Dietary fiber prefers not to leave without first making some important chemical connections.

So why—with such great differences—are both types called fiber? Because both are "waste," indigestible residue that does not get absorbed by the blood.

Your next question: Then why is any of it, regardless of type, so important?

Studies have shown that fiber can relieve constipation problems by absorbing water and hence adding size and softness to feces. And studies also suggest that fiber may be able to prevent appendicitis, hemorrhoids, diverticulosis, cardiovascular disease, and cancer of the colon.

But to enjoy the full range of fiber's benefits, it is best to draw from a wide range of sources. With fiber, different types appear to be more suited to different gripes.

The bullish fibers (cellulose and lignin) in whole wheat products, for example, are better at providing stool bulk than are the more minute pectic substances in vegetables and fruits. But then, vegetables and fruits seem better at supervising the cleanliness of the blood.

When raw carrots were fed to a group of men along with their normal breakfast, their cholesterol levels dropped by an average of 11 percent in just three weeks. Similar cholesterol-lowering effects, however, have *not* been found to occur in response to diets rich solely in wheat products or bran.

Why?

Because the primary function of the relatively large and abrasive fibers in wheat products and bran is to provide stool bulk by absorbing water, and to speed transit time as a result. This effect may discourage cholesterol absorption in the intestine somewhat, but scientists are finding that fruits and vegetables are better suited for this because of their higher pectin content.

Pectin discourages cholesterol absorption on a *chemical* level—by rendering bile acids (responsible for breaking cholesterol down into absorbable form) inactive.

What this suggests is that the best approach to fiber is to enjoy the best of both worlds: whole wheat products, whole grain cereals, and bran for rapid elimination; fruits and vegetables for insuring that these fast-moving stools take with them their share of cholesterol.

The sanitizing effects of a diet well balanced in fiber, however, do not stop here—because it's felt that the same bile acids that encourage cholesterol absorption may also encourage cancer in the colon.

"Some of the bile acids in men have been shown to be promoters of cancer in experimental animals," reports Jon A. Story, Ph.D., of the Department of Foods and Nutrition at Purdue University. Fiber, by flushing the intestines clean of these potentially damaging acids, "appears to hold great potential," Dr. Story says, for affording protection against this disease.

Fiber, as you can see, is more than just a laxative; it's a type of internal detergent. So now the question: How much do I need to keep myself a clean machine?

Not to depress you, but if you eat like most Americans, you would do well to get about five times as much fiber as you do. Most authorities agree that something in the neighborhood of 20 grams of dietary fiber a day is what your body—by design—should get.

Does that mean you start dusting your every bite with wheat bran?

No. It means you start increasing both the quantity *and the variety* of fiber in your diet by tapping all available sources—not just the obvious ones like whole grains, beans, and vegetables, but also such *un*likely ones as bananas, blackberries, and peanut butter. Not all types, remember, go crunch.

Take a look at the preceding table. We've done our best to enrich it with foods that, in addition to being fibrous, are also fun.

20/
Why You Should
Eat More Oxygen

You could live for about two months without food and about three days without water. But you could live for only about six minutes without oxygen. It's very important stuff—and not just for your lungs.

Every cell in your body needs oxygen constantly. Without it, the trillions of chemical reactions that go on inside you every second would come to a halt. And you would die.

So how healthy can it be to eat foods that prevent oxygen from moving as freely through your body as it should?

That's the question that Don Mannerberg, M.D. (former medical director of the Cooper Aerobics Center in Dallas), asks in his book *Aerobic Nutrition* (E. P. Dutton, 1981). Dr. Mannerberg maintains that the standard American diet impedes the transport of oxygen to cells by overloading the blood with fat.

"Most people assume that as long as they are breathing in air, their bodies will get as much oxygen as they need," Dr. Mannerberg says. But that air "may never get very far beyond the lungs.

"It's supposed to be delivered throughout the body by a remarkable system of red blood cell carriers. But when people follow a diet of high fat content, concentrated sugars, and too much alcohol, triglycerides reach high levels in the blood and cause the red blood cells to clump together." This clumping, Dr. Mannerberg asserts, can lead to problems in two ways.

First, it gives oxygen molecules less surface area to cling to, thus reducing the oxygen-carrying capacity of the blood; and second, it slows the flow of blood through the smallest of our blood vessels, the capillaries. "This particularly affects vital organs such as the brain, liver, and kidneys," Dr. Mannerberg says, which are not muscular and so cannot be given oxygen by way of exercise.

The result?

"Partial starvation of oxygen and nutrients eventually produces degenerative diseases: heart disease, diabetes, atherosclerosis, malfunctioning gallbladder, and so on. Instead of blooming, the total body begins to wilt."

It's not a pretty picture that the doctor paints. Can our scrumptious breakfasts of bacon and eggs really be that bad?

Dr. Mannerberg's argument relies as much on theory as it does on clinical proof, but it warrants consideration nonetheless. It is not known for sure that high triglycerides lead to the deterioration of vital organs, but it is known that they're a risk factor for heart disease. And whether or not sugar and fat wind up shortchanging us of oxygen, they *do* wind up shortchanging us of vitamins, minerals, protein, and fiber. And that *is* something to gasp about.

Currently the average American diet derives about 42 percent of its calories from fat and another 17 percent from refined sugars. Toss in about 7 percent from alcohol and you're looking at a diet that offers 66 percent—two-thirds—of its calories in forms that are virtually devoid of nutrients. Add a pack of cigarettes to that diet and you've really got something to choke on.

Why?

Because the inhalation of tobacco smoke *has* been shown to reduce oxygen levels in the blood, first by decreasing the amount of oxygen that lungs can absorb because of tar buildup, and then by reducing the oxygen-carrying capacity of red blood cells by tying them up with carbon monoxide. If that's not enough, nicotine has been shown to constrict capillaries, thus reducing the flow of blood that is short of oxygen in the first place.

So whether or not Dr. Mannerberg's attack on our eating habits is squarely on target, his assault on our smoking habits is. And he also makes some good points about our activity levels. Perhaps the *best* way to satisfy the body's appetite for oxygen, he says, is to breathe. The more the better. Breathing doesn't have to be heavy—just as long as it's often.

"The key word is motion," Dr. Mannerberg feels. Take stairs instead of elevators; arrange your office conveniently so that you have to get up a lot; retire your gardener. The more movement you can put into your life, the better—because movement of *any* kind requires the intake of more oxygen than remaining stationary.

And as a plus for you weight watchers, oxygen doesn't have any calories. In fact, oxygen burns calories. Recent studies done by scientists at the University of New Hampshire suggest that the more oxygen your muscles are capable of using, the less chance you have of putting on fat.

And how do you improve the ability of your muscles to process oxygen?

The concept of getting more oxygen into one's life is an interesting way of looking at the pursuit of health. Because if it's true that healthful foods are better at keeping optimum supplies of oxygen in our blood—and that abstinence from smoking and getting daily exercise also are important—the quest for oxygen constitutes a total health package. The diet Dr. Mannerberg recommends is low in fat and sugar and high in complex carbohydrates and fiber. The rest of his program encourages regular daily exercise, straightforward dealings with stress, and moderation in the use of alcohol. The program, in fact, comes very close to that of Nathan Pritikin, which is understandable considering that Dr. Mannerberg served as director of medical services at the Pritikin Longevity Center in California.

Can this program work?

That depends on what you mean by work. We're not going to promise that chasing after oxygen is going to have you doing wind sprints at 100. But if it's more energy, less body fat, and lower blood fats you're after, we'd say Dr. Mannerberg's program of "aerobic nutrition" can have you on the right track.

Basic Tenets of "Aerobic Nutrition"

- Reduce total fat intake to no more than 20 percent of your total caloric intake. (This requires cutting down on butter, oleomargarine, vegetable shortening, cooking and salad oils, whole milk products, cheese, and fatty meats.)
- Increase consumption of fruits, vegetables, and complex

Why the Move to More Chicken and Fish

It's getting as trendy among the health conscious as having mineral water instead of a cocktail—fish and fowl instead of beef. Ever wonder why?

Perhaps the biggest problem with the typical American diet, as Don Mannerberg, M.D., points out, is the amount of fat it contains. Directly, that high fat content has been linked with coronary heart disease and cancers of the breast and colon; indirectly—by making us obese—it has been blamed as a contributor to high blood pressure, hardening of the arteries, gallbladder disease, liver disease, and diabetes.

Fat, though, comes in three forms—not all of which are thought to be equally hazardous to our health.

Saturated fats (most common in foods of animal origin) are considered the most dangerous because they can raise the amount of cholesterol in our blood.

Monounsaturated fats (found mostly in plant foods, but also in some animal products) do not appear to affect cholesterol levels either way.

Polyunsaturated fats (found in plant and animal foods) have an ability to *lower* serum cholesterol levels. Polyunsaturated fats, moreover, are the only kind our bodies need because only they contain linoleic acid, a substance necessary for the health of our cell membranes. The other kinds of fat we *could* do without.

Back to chicken and fish.

In addition to containing less total fat, they also contain less of the bad, and more of the better, two varieties of unsaturated fat: mono- and poly- (see accompanying table).

Our goal should be to reduce our fat intake across the board, because all types are equally high in calories. But the idea behind the chicken and fish movement is to get less of the saturated, and more of the mono- and polyunsaturated types.

carbohydrates (starches) preferably in the form of whole grain breads, brown rice, potatoes, and beans.
- Reduce consumption of sugar, jams, and syrups.
- Eat eggs sparingly.
- Make chicken and fish (baked or broiled) your primary sources of meat.
- Reduce salt intake.
- Get moderate daily exercise.
- Go easy on alcohol.
- Learn to deal with stress.
- Don't smoke.

Types of Fat in Selected Meats, Poultry, and Fish

	Portion (ounces)	Saturated Fat (grams)	Monoun- saturated Fat (grams)	Polyun- saturated Fat (grams)	Protein (grams)	Calories
Sirloin steak, broiled	3	13.1	12.0	0.5	19.6	329
Veal, rib, roasted	3	6.9	6.3	0.3	23.1	229
Beef liver, fried, no added fat	3½	1.8	0.7	0.7	22.9	149
Ham, light cure, roasted	3	6.8	7.9	1.7	17.8	246
Pork loin, fresh, roasted	3	8.7	10.2	2.2	20.8	308
Chicken, flesh only, broiled	3½	1.3	1.5	0.8	23.8	136
Chicken liver, simmered	3½	1.8	1.3	0.9	18.6	116
Turkey: dark meat, roasted	3	2.0	3.0	1.5	25.5	173
light meat, roasted	3	1.0	1.4	0.7	28.0	150
Haddock, raw	3½	0.12	0.09	0.19	18.3	79
Tuna: canned in oil, drained	3	1.7	1.7	0.7	24.0	170
canned in water	3½	0.22	0.15	0.23	28.0	127
Cod, raw	3½	0.13	0.09	0.28	17.6	82
Flounder, raw	3½	3.3	0.3	0.40	16.7	82
Sole, raw	3½	0.16	0.1	0.30	16.7	78

SOURCES: U.S. Department of Agriculture Handbook nos. 8 and 456; *Nutritive Value of Foods*, Home and Garden Bulletin no. 72, by Catherine F. Adams and Martha Richardson (Washington, D.C.: Science and Education Administration, U.S. Department of Agriculture, 1978); and USDA Nutrient Data Research Group, 1981.

21/

Foods That Can Heal

Scientists are finally getting around to realizing what witch doctors and grandmothers have known all along: There are foods that can heal.

"Beyond any doubt," says V. Petkov, Ph.D., D.Sc., of the Bulgarian Academy of Sciences, "the plant world represents an inexhaustible source of chemical compounds, many of them having high biological activity."

Soybeans, garlic, cranberries, watercress, cabbage, and carrots—scientists are discovering healing powers in these foods that could have the prescription of the future looking like a grocery list.

And why not? It was, after all, from plants that man got the idea of medicine in the first place. Your doctor may not be eager to admit it, but many of the drugs being prescribed today are little more than synthetic versions of things that two thousand years ago might have been given to you as a soup.

Aspirin, for example, is a chemical copy of a time-proven painkiller first found centuries ago in the leaves and bark of the willow. The method of modern pharmacology, basically, has been to isolate, imitate, and then increase the potency of chemical compounds that Mother Nature (perhaps more wisely) saw fit to keep relatively dilute in the presence of other ingredients. As Andrew Weil, M.D., a research associate at the Harvard Botanical Museum, explains it, "Plants with medicinal properties are complex mixtures of things. One chemical may be principally responsible for an effect, but other secondary components may be just as important as modifiers of this effect. With a plant drug, there is an interaction of a variety of compounds that makes it safer and more effective."

And more confusing. If the scientific community has been reluctant to pursue herbal medicine, it has been as much out of frustration as disrespect.

Recently, however, there has been a renewed interest in folk medicine—foods in particular. Influenced partially by the impasse that the drug industry has reached in its attempts to arrest our two worst killers—heart disease and cancer—some researchers have been turning their microscopes "back to nature" to see what a more organic approach may have to offer. And what they've been finding has been encouraging.

The wisdom of herbal medicine, herbalists say, is that it helps our bodies help themselves. By enhancing rather than usurping the powers of our immune systems, medicines that occur naturally are thought to be able to "fix" things as they were meant to be fixed: slowly, as the saying goes, but surely. Modern medicines, natural healers complain, focus on symptoms at the expense of their causes.

This is, after all, the easier way. What has kept the likes of garlic off your physician's prescription list has been the intricacy—and, unfortunately, mystery—behind the way it works. It is much easier and safer for your doctor to deal with drugs whose effects and appropriate dosages he knows precisely. With plants, whose potencies can vary by as much as 60 percent due to climatic conditions alone, the science of writing out prescriptions comes apart at the seams.

Despite this disadvantage, however, naturally occurring medicines offer amazing potential. Take a look at the following review we've made of the most noteworthy studies done on such cures to date. If our accounts of the exact mechanisms by which these cures work seem sketchy, it's because what scientists have been able to determine is sketchy. Consider this element of uncertainty as testimony to the level of complexity on which these cures function.

Chicken Soup and the Common Cold

Yes, hot chicken soup can help cure a cold. The reason it can, doctors from Mount Sinai Medical Center in Miami Beach say, is that it reduces the amount of time that germ-infested mucus stays in contact with nasal passages (i.e., it makes your nose run). Researchers pitted chicken soup against hot water in an experiment designed to measure the velocity of mucus transport. While hot water could speed mucus along (from 6.2 millimeters per minute to 8.4 millimeters per minute), chicken soup was able to get it up to 9.2 millimeters per minute. That's important, the researchers say, because colds often linger due to sluggish mucus transport.

The precise mechanism responsible for this power of chicken soup was not, however, determined. It's partially due to its warmth, partially to its aroma, and partially to some other "mechanism related to taste," is all the director of Mount Sinai's medical services, Marvin Sackner, M.D., could say (*Chest*, October, 1978).

Garlic for Healthier Blood

Forgetting, for the time being, healing claims an herbalist might make (for example, rheumatism, asthma, epilepsy, dementia, constipation, ailing internal organs, and a slipping sex life), what garlic *can* fix, according to a study done in India, is high levels of fat in the blood. When doctors at the B. J. Medical College and Sassoon General Hospitals in Pune, India, studied lovers, haters, and takers-or-leavers of garlic, they found that the blood fat levels of these three groups varied *in direct proportion* to their fondness for the herb.

Additional research has led scientists to believe that garlic further improves blood by increasing what they call fibrinolytic activity—the ability of the blood to resist clotting. In one experiment, the fibrinolytic activity of heart attack patients increased by 95 percent in just 20 days when they were fed garlic oil. (In a group of normal people, fibrinolytic activity increased by 130 percent when they were fed the oil.) These findings have led researchers to believe that garlic has great potential for lessening the chances of further attacks in people who have suffered myocardial infarctions. The researcher who conducted the study, Dr. Arun Bordia of the R. N. T. Medical College in Udaipur, India, concluded, "The herbal remedy has proven effective, clinically acceptable, and safe" (*Atherosclerosis,* October, 1977).

Soybeans for Cholesterol, Cancer, and Tooth Decay

Soybeans, at times, seem just too good to be true. Nutritionally, they're about as complete as a food can be. Now it's being found that they're not too bad at playing doctor, either.

When a team of scientists at the University of Milan in Italy fed soybeans to adults with high levels of cholesterol, they were surprised to find that cholesterol levels dropped by more than 20 percent. In the words of one of the researchers, "The cholesterol-lowering effect exhibited by the soybean diet was remarkable; it was achieved within a few weeks and was probably superior to that expected even from several months' treatment with a low-fat diet" (*Lancet,* January 19, 1980).

Against cancer, the soybean may not be as effective—but it shows promise nonetheless. Walter Troll, Ph.D., of the New York University Medical Center, has been able to isolate a "protease inhibitor" in soy protein that he feels may counteract certain enzymes responsible for tumor growth.

Tooth decay? Evidence here comes from Dr. Takeo Shiozawa, director of the Masago Dental Clinic in Japan. Dr. Shiozawa compared the effects of a high-soybean diet to a high-milk diet in rats and found, surprisingly, that the rats reared on soybeans were far more resistant to tooth decay (when made to eat sugar) than the milk-fed rats. Dr. Shiozawa credits glycine—an amino acid in soybeans—for these results.

Yogurt for Cholesterol

If there's any truth to Dannon's claim that yogurt can keep you as spry as a Soviet Georgian, it may hinge on yogurt's recently discovered ability to lower cholesterol. When doctors from Harbor/University of California at Los Angeles General Hospital fed yogurt to 54 healthy subjects, they found that their serum cholesterol levels dropped between 5 and 10 percent within seven days.

Researchers feel that several factors may have been responsible for these results. Yogurt contains large amounts of calcium, which is known to block cholesterol absorption in the intestine. And yogurt also contains a substance (hydroxymethyl glutarate) which some researchers feel discourages cholesterol synthesis. As for any part played by live cultures in yogurt, researchers were forced to dismiss this possibility when yogurt *not* containing cultures proved to lower cholesterol also (*American Journal of Clinical Nutrition,* January, 1979).

Raw Cabbage for Ulcers

In a study done by a team of doctors from University College Hospital Medical School in London, rats were fed various diets to test the effects of certain foods suspected of protecting against ulcers. The foods tested were lettuce, milk powder, lentils, wheat bran, polished and unpolished rice, a grain and vegetable from India, and cabbage.

After every imaginable combination of these foods was tried, it became clear that the vegetables were better protectors than the grains, and that the best of the vegetables was cabbage—raw. (Its effectiveness was reduced substantially when cooked.)

Why did some foods work better than others?

The researchers suggest that the foods not only minimized the amount of potentially harmful acids, but also buffered the stomach against them (*Postgraduate Medicine,* June, 1975).

Fruits and Vegetables for Obesity and Constipation

That may sound like a tall order, but when 12 men (aged 35 to 49) were fed a diet rich in fruits and vegetables for a period of 21 days, they experienced larger, more frequent bowel movements, and their fecal matter contained more fat (meaning the men, as a result, retained less).

Why?

Fiber. As we've already pointed out, a diet rich in fruits and vegetables offers several kinds: cellulose and hemicellulose (which also occur in wheat bran), and pectin (a kind found only in fruit). Cellulose and hemicellulose encourage stool frequency and weight, while pectin increases excretion of fat —by binding fat with bile acids, making fat difficult for the intestines to absorb.

Fish for the Blood

Forget the brain; fish can fix your blood. When 19 volunteers from a monastery and 23 from a convent took part in an experiment designed to test the fat-lowering effects of fish, 200 grams (about seven ounces) of mackerel a day for three weeks produced the following results: Serum cholesterol levels dropped by an average of 7.5 percent; serum triglycerides (another undesirable fat) dropped an average of 35 percent; HDL cholesterol (the good kind) went up in the men (but not in the women); and very-low-density cholesterol or VLDL (a bad kind) went down in everybody (*American Journal of Clinical Nutrition*, August, 1978).

Why these dramatic results?

The researchers in charge of the study could not say.

Vegetables against Cancer

Studies here are still in a preliminary stage, but what's been found so far looks encouraging: Juices from some very common vegetables have been found to reduce the cell mutations produced by carcinogens in tobacco smoke and burned meat.

Dr. Tsuneo Kada, a mutation specialist working at the National Institute of Genetics in Japan, discovered that juices made from various raw vegetables (cabbage, lettuce, cauliflower, radish, turnip, asparagus, bean sprouts, and peas) substantially reduced the mutagenic activity of the nitrosamines that he mixed with these juices in a vial. Dr. Kada suspects that enzymes in the vegetables were responsible, because cooking noticeably reduced their effectiveness.

An Overview

Should these recent findings affect the way you eat?

Absolutely. Because as good as these foods are at healing, they're even better at prevention. More fruits, vegetables, fiber-rich whole grain products, low-fat dairy products, soy proteins, chicken, and fish. Less fatty meats, highly processed foods, and sugar. By eating more of the foods that heal—and less of those that hurt—you offer health a fighting chance, and maybe even a victory.

SECTION II/EXERCISE

I got to thinking the other night what might make for the ideal "high." It would have to be something that:

A. made us feel good
B. about ourselves
C. in a way that was also good for us.

I came up with exercise.

22/
Why Exercise Doesn't Have to Be Hard

Have you ever wondered what sort of shape our prehistoric ancestors were in?

It matters, because if they were slouches, then maybe we can be, too. After all, part of the logic behind exercise is that it re-creates some of the physical conditions under which we evolved. And if those conditions were duck soup, then it would follow that we—in our running shoes—are perhaps overstepping our evolutionary limits.

We asked an anthropologist about it. And from what Vaughn Bryant, Ph.D., head of the Department of Anthropology at Texas A & M University, has been able to determine, the caveman (sorry, sedentaries) was a veritable dynamo.

"We were working at a site in Texas, doing exploratory digging in caves where these people had lived, set on the side of a canyon wall," Dr. Bryant told us. "Talk about a climb. There were 19 of us, 12 of whom couldn't make it. A climb that prehistoric man was making every day—like taking out the garbage—and 12 modern young people, college kids, couldn't even make it—once!"

What does this tell us about the caveman's fitness program? That it achieved phenomenal results. Naturally.

"Exercise for these people was a way of life," Dr. Bryant said. "It is unlikely that they ever really pushed themselves. But then, getting the amount of exercise they did—all day, every day—they didn't have to.

"We estimate that on a hunt, prehistoric man might have covered about 10 miles, routinely. And the women and children, whose job it was to gather most of the plant foods, probably went between four and six, every day."

"Running?" we asked.

"No. Walking," he said. "The men might have jogged at certain times during their hunts, but primarily these ventures were exercises in tracking." As for the women and children, "they were gathering things, remember," Dr. Bryant said. "Running would have been inappropriate, to say the least."

Inappropriate. If that's what running, or weight training, or calisthenics have been for you, then take heart in the caveman's tale. He did not jog on his lunch hour, or pump iron at the Y, or do jumping jacks along with Jack LaLanne, and yet "he was an extremely muscular being," Dr. Bryant said, "with bones, tendons, and ligaments much more rugged than our own." Fred Flintstone, Dr. Bryant feels, would have made a very good linebacker.

Does this mean that the way we approach fitness—in bursts—goes for naught as we sit back down at our desks to make our livings?

No. It simply means that these bursts are not the only way, that every little

Down with the Elevator—Take the Stairs

If you either work or live on a floor higher than the thirteenth, you're in luck: Fitness for you is as easy as never having to wait for another elevator.

In a study done by an insurance company in Finland, a "significant level of fitness" was achieved by men who were made to climb an average of 25 flights of stairs a day. In a world of skyscrapers, that's not a lot.

Roy Shepard, M.D., professor of applied physiology at the University of Toronto, has determined that a sedentary person who climbs a flight of nine-inch steps at 30 to 40 steps per minute uses about 50 percent of his maximum oxygen uptake. This degree of exertion, moreover, escalates rather quickly. Studies done by cardiologists Lenore R. Zohman, M.D., and Albert A. Kattus, M.D., show that a stair-climber's heart rate goes up about ten beats for every flight (*The Cardiologist's Guide to Fitness and Health through Exercise*, Simon and Schuster, 1979). So if your pulse is 70 at rest, six flights of stairs (consisting of eight to ten eight-inch steps per flight) would have you ticking along at about 130 by the time you got done—a figure well within the target exercise heart rate (the rate that produces a training effect) for most people.

Coming down is no cake walk, either. Drs. Zohman and Kattus have determined that it's one-third to one-half as hard as going up.

Calories burned climbing?

Monumental—over 1,000 an hour for a large man. You can figure your own rate (per minute of stair climbing) by dividing your body weight by 22. (A man or woman weighing 154 pounds, for example, burns about seven calories a minute.) Pace, for the purpose of this calculation, is taken to be what Drs. Zohman and Kattus call "comfortable"—slightly less than two steps per second, or about five seconds per average eight to ten steps. By taking steps two at a time, calorie consumption more than doubles.

So stop waiting for elevators. Dr. Shepard claims that a program of climbing three flights of stairs in succession (in 30 seconds or less) nine to ten times a day can get you in shape.

bit of exercise we get throughout our lives may be as important as the miles we log daily.

A tribe that lives today in the Himalaya mountains much as the caveman did millions of years ago would seem to bear this out. These people (the Hunzas) commonly live to be more than 120 years old, but they take no formal exercise. Working on their terraced farm fields from sunrise to sunset, they get all the exercise they need the way the caveman did—naturally.

Perhaps the way we should, too. Not that high-intensity exercises such as fast running, hard cycling, and weight lifting are bad—just concentrated, much like our modern-day approach to healing in general. When we want health, we want it in a hurry. And so with our exercise, as with our drugs, we suffer our share of side effects (pulled muscles and shin splints) accordingly. By comparison, it is unlikely that many cave people were sidelined by runner's knee.

Exercise, quite simply, does not have to be hard in order to be good for you. It has to be hard if you want to be an Olympic champion, but it does not have to be hard if you just want to be healthy. Some very interesting studies have been done with heart attack patients recently to bear this out.

When 32 victims (aged 35 to 68) of myocardial infarction, for example, were put on a 13-week walking program (which progressed to slow jogging only if participants felt up to it), researchers observed a marked increase in their HDL. (HDL, remember, is a blood component that helps protect against heart disease by clearing excess cholesterol out of the bloodstream.) Circulating insulin levels in these men also took a turn for the better (they went down). The amount of exercise responsible for these results was a modest mile and three-quarters of walking/jogging three times a week (*Journal of the American Medical Association*, November 16, 1979).

In another study published in the same journal, similar results were achieved when 83 heart attack patients were made to exercise lightly for 45 minutes, three times a week. This program involved slow jogging interspersed with walking and light calisthenics, and even though few of the participants —even after six months—had progressed beyond a modest mile and a half of very slow running three times a week, their HDL levels had increased by an average of about 14 percent. These results prompted the study's director, D. Willem Erkelens, M.D., to conclude with some surprise that the "amount of exercise needed to increase HDL levels does not appear to be very great."

Endocrinologist Dan Streja, M.D., of California agrees. "To favorably alter cholesterol, to lower blood sugar, insulin, and triglyceride levels, and to lose weight, walking will do it," Dr. Streja told us. "Metabolically speaking, walking is as good as running."

If those words—"metabolically speaking"—sound like a monumental concession, they're not. Unless you're exercising to excel athletically, metabolics are all you really need to worry about. Yes, high-intensity exercise increases HDL more than low-intensity exercise, but not by much. And it is unlikely that this marginal difference is worth the monumental strain, particularly if this strain is going to discourage you from exercising in the first place.

That's the bottom line: exercising in the first place. As Charles T. Kuntzleman, Ed.D., author of *The Complete Book of Walking* (Simon and Schuster, 1978), puts it, "You can't get benefits from any exercise you don't do."

If you're on a tight schedule, and you find that quick half-hour jogs suit it, fine. For its sheer convenience and physiologic efficiency, running is probably the best exercise you can do. Swimming, cross-country skiing, and cycling also are excellent overall conditioners. But . . .

They are concentrated. More concentrated, perhaps, than you—if your history has been sedentary—would prefer.

Exercise, in short, need not be an all-or-nothing affair. There are many valuable levels in between. Evolution was five million years in putting us together—not as marathoners or weight lifters or swimmers of the English Channel, but rather as walkers. And as workers. Certainly you can find the energy to be a combination of those.

23/

Eight Reasons Not to Exercise—
All of Them Wrong

Roughly half the adult population is now exercising with some regularity. Which leaves roughly half who are not. What excuses do these holdouts have?

Some doozies. Several years ago a Harris Poll was conducted to get an idea of these excuses; what emerged as the most popular are the erroneous notions listed below. Are you fit enough to defend yours?

1. *I get enough exercise around the house.* Must be some house. Unless you're getting at least 15 minutes of nonstop exercise three times a week, you're not getting enough.
2. *After a long day at work, I don't have the energy to exercise.* Baloney. That's when you need to exercise most, to get a "second wind" for a productive evening. Exercise can *give* you energy.
3. *Exercise will increase my appetite and make me overeat.* Not true. Exercise has been shown to be an appetite "equalizer." Overweight people tend to eat *less* when they exercise.
4. *Fads about fitness come and go.* Since when? You're confusing fitness with the hula hoop. Surveys predict a slight leveling off of the current running craze, but the interest in fitness in general, they say, is here to stay.
5. *Too much exercise will enlarge my heart, which can be bad if I stop.* Congratulations—you're only half wrong. Exercise makes your heart a bigger (and better) muscle, which will simply return to its original size if you quit.
6. *Middle-aged and older people don't need anything more than a little stretching.* Sorry, old-timer. The body is a muscle, born to be worked. And it dies as fast as we let it. Studies have shown that vigorous exercise firms bones and strengthens skin.
7. *The trouble with participating in a sport is that I can only get to it now and then, and I hear that too much exertion at one time*

can be bad. That's true, so find a sport you can play regularly. You don't need to go anywhere to jump rope.

8. *Too many people, such as joggers and weight lifters, become fanatical about fitness.* Stand up and say that! True, some people get carried away—but the dangers of doing too much are far less than doing too little.

24/

Exercise and the Aging Process

As a kid, Jack LaLanne was downright sickly. He wore arch supports, a back brace, and glasses. Then Jack found exercise. And the impish muscle man has had Father Time in a half nelson ever since.

To celebrate his sixty-fifth birthday, Jack tugged 65 boats loaded with 65,000 pounds of wood pulp 1½ miles across Lake Osuoku in Tokyo with hands cuffed and feet tied.

Why?

"To prove that as we get older, we don't have to dissipate and wither," Jack said.

The medical world is beginning to agree. According to C. Carson Conrad, executive director of the President's Council on Physical Fitness and Sports, "A scientific breakthrough of major significance has been the recognition that many problems long attributed to aging are, in fact, infirmities that could be avoided if people would only be more active."

What sort of infirmities?

The kind you've been dreading: reduced muscle strength, shortness of breath, slowed reflexes, soft bones, stiffness, senility, and a double chin. That may sound like a tough bill to fill, but it's not.

Exercise works its rejuvenatory magic by making us breathe. Doctors call the process "maximal oxygen uptake," and what it does—on a molecular level —is infuse our bodies' cells with oxygen. Studies have shown that after the age of about 20, when many of us begin to get lazy, we process about 1 percent less oxygen every year. The result of this cutback is a commensurate decline in cellular activity. Our bodies, in a sense, begin to suffocate.

Exercise can prevent this by keeping heart and lungs strong enough to supply the amounts of oxygen our bodies grew up with. Studies have shown that people who remain active as they get older—*very* active—can maintain breathing capacities equal to people *40 years* their junior.

The effects of this kind of youthful oxygen supply are far-reaching, as the following studies will show. What's more, they can be achieved at nearly any age. Physiologists in one experiment found that a group of previously unconditioned men and women—*aged 60 to 83*—were able to improve their breathing capacities by 29 percent in a year's time simply by doing light calisthenics and walking. This gain, the researchers said, compared very favorably to what might have been expected from people much younger.

The other side of the hill, in other words, doesn't have to be a cliff. Take a look at the following evidence. In the words of Theodore Klumpp, M.D. (a medical consultant to the President's Council on Physical Fitness and Sports), "Staying active is the key to staying alive."

Heart and Lungs

Many people think of their bodies as machines composed of parts that wear out. Not so.

Our bodies *respond* to physical stress by adapting and growing stronger. This response is what evolution, and survival, is all about. And it holds true for more than just our muscles.

Heart and lungs, for example. They don't get tired as we get older, they get lazy. A team of doctors from the Washington School of Medicine in St. Louis proved this recently by comparing two groups of middle-aged men on an exercise treadmill. They found that a group of runners (average age 58) had cardiovascular systems *twice* as capable as a group of sedentaries whose average age was 54 (*Journal of Applied Physiology*, vol. 51, no. 3, 1981).

The heart, we seem to forget, is a muscle—and needs to be exercised accordingly.

Bones

Few people think of bones as living tissue, but they are. And they respond to environmental stress (exercise) accordingly. As bones get stressed by the muscular contractions and compressional impacts of exercise, they respond by taking on more calcium and phosphorus—getting thicker, denser, and stronger as a result.

"A physical activity lifestyle above a sedentary level is needed to induce
. . this calcification," say two doctors reporting in *Nutrition Reports International* (June, 1978). "[Bone] growth and increase in the density of the bone occur in proportion to the compressional load a bone is asked to carry."

Skin

Forget the face-lift. A better way of ironing out the wrinkles—or preventing them, anyway—could be to get fit. A team of doctors from Finland has found that what makes your face red—oxygen—also makes it rugged.

These doctors took skin samples from the upper arm of 29 athletic middle-aged men and compared them with similar samples taken from 29 sedentaries.

The difference, they found, was that the skin of the athletes—in this case, runners and cross-country skiers (good for 30 miles a week)—was thicker and more elastic than the skin of their less active peers.

Why?

"The results suggest that skin reflects an adaptation to habitual endurance training by increasing its mass and strengthening its structure," the researchers said (*British Journal of Dermatology,* August, 1978).

Brain

Last, but not least—the oxygen that exercise pumps to your body is also pumped to your head. And the effects of this supply over the years, scientists are finding, appear to be substantial.

Perhaps the best example of exercise's effects on cerebral functioning comes from two researchers from San Diego State University who tested the cognitive reaction times of 64 men and women (aged 23 to 59), half of whom were habitual runners, the other half sedentaries.

What was tested was how fast each participant could react to an electric stimulus by releasing either his right or left index finger from a switch. (If this seems like a crude measure of mental aging, it is not. "Cognitive reaction times provide an excellent indication of how effectively and efficiently the processes of the central nervous system are working," the researchers said, "and are often used to measure degrees of senility for this reason.")

Results surprised even the researchers. The group of nonrunners demonstrated slowed reaction times consistent with their age. The runners, on the other hand, showed no slowdown whatsoever (*Medicine and Science in Sports,* vol. 11, no. 2, 1979).

Exercise, then, seems to strengthen nerve tissue in much the same way as it does muscles. The increased enzyme activity and abundant blood flow caused by exercise appear to safeguard the overall health of the central nervous system—brain included.

Jack LaLanne has been doing push-ups ever since his teens. Eighty-year-old national Amateur Athletic Union track champion Paul Spangler, on the other hand, didn't start exercising until the ripe age of 67.

It really *is* never too late.

If Not Longer, Certainly Better

Evidence that physical exercise can help us live longer is scant. Perhaps the most convincing, in fact, comes to us only by way of a study done with rats in which a group of exercised females outlived a group of sedentaries by 11.5 percent, and a group of exercised males outlived their restricted counterparts by 19.3 percent (*Gerontology,* January, 1980). For humans, we can only turn to the examples put forth by population studies showing that physical activity and longevity *seem* to go hand in hand.

Before you toss in the towel, though, consider this: There is no doubt —even among normally very objective scientists—that exercise can help us live *better.*

At a nutrition conference presented by the Boston University School of Medicine, Michael Klein, M.D., reported on the effects of a ten-week (thrice-weekly) aerobic exercise program on 65 male corporate executives (average age 45). And, of course, dramatic physical improvements were made: Cholesterol levels, body fat percentages, diastolic blood pressures, heart rates, body weights, HDL cholesterol levels, and maximal oxygen uptakes all took turns for the better. But . . .

Less predictable were the *mental* gains made by these men. Psychological examinations revealed that they were less tense, anxious, and hostile, and that they reported feeling less stress following the ten-week exercise experience.

As Walter M. Bortz, M.D., put it in the *Journal of the American Geriatrics Society* (February, 1980), "For both the ill and the healthy, a vigorous activity pattern seems to confer manifold advantages for the mind, body, and possibly most importantly, the spirit. . . ."

It's nice to know that the medical community is finally catching on to what the athletic community has known all along: Fitness *feels* good.

25/
How to Improve Your Relationship with Exercise

Getting involved with exercise is a little like getting married: It's easy enough in the beginning because it's novel—but the initial attraction has a way of wearing thin. If you are currently betrothed to an exercise program, be totally honest and answer the following questions:

- Do you hate waking up to it in the morning?
- Do you dread coming home to it at night?
- Is it causing you pain?
- Are you cheating on it?

If so, you're in need of counseling. Because, as we pointed out in the last chapter, it's important that you and exercise stick together—*forever.* Exercise, in fact, is like security in the sense that it becomes more important the older we get.

So take a look at the following six categories that describe your relationship with exercise. And be sincere in deciding which best applies to you. Five out of the six entail their own special set of problems—which *can,* however, be worked out. With a little bit of effort, there's no reason you can't improve your relationship with exercise immensely . . . maybe even to the point of being with it "till death do you part."

Complete this sentence: My relationship with exercise can best be described as:

A. nonexistent.
B. occasional and begrudging.
C. occasional and loving.
D. regular but begrudging.
E. regular and loving.
F. compulsive and sometimes injurious to my health.

A. Nonexistent

If you've yet to flirt with exercise, your chances of entering into a lasting relationship with it are actually quite good, for several reasons.

First off, because you are mature, you will no doubt approach exercise in a mature and sensible fashion. Secondly, the positive feelings you get from exercise as a middle-aged "single" are apt to come as a welcome cure for the midlife blahs. And finally, with no history of former athletic greatness to haunt you, you are going to be able to view your efforts as part of an *upward* rather than a downward swing.

B. Occasional and Begrudging

Your problem with exercise is that you make it too hard on yourself. You either try to do too much at once (like squeezing a week's worth of running into a Saturday) or you exercise for the wrong reasons (to cure hangovers or burn off banana splits). No wonder it's no fun.

What should you do?

Make exercise easier to live with. And stop using it as a form of punishment. Start thinking frequency rather than intensity; pleasure rather than pain. Laboratory experiments have shown that three times a week, easy, confers more benefits than once a week, hard. And keep in mind, too, that exercise is not the great eraser of evils that you think it is. You'd have to run about 11 miles to burn off half a fifth of scotch. And you'd still have done nothing to patch things up with your liver.

C. Occasional and Loving

Your problem with exercise is that you like it too much: those romantic games of golf (played once a week) that finish up on the eighteenth green precisely at sunset; the tennis dates that are almost too much fun to take time off from work to keep. Exercise for you is a form of indulgence, something you feel guilty about taking the time to do.

Well, don't. Because it's more important than you're giving it credit for. You should be doing something physical *three times* a week, for at least 20 minutes at a time. And at the risk of spoiling your love affair with golf, it wouldn't be a bad idea to *work* a bit during those 20 minutes. Would you be as infatuated with the links, for that matter, if you and your clubs could not be chauffeured about in a cart? Exercise should be fun, but not a bed of roses.

D. Regular but Begrudging

Your trouble is that you have a distorted idea of what exercise should be, and you always have, right from the time you were made to run wind sprints (ad nauseam) to show how much you wanted to play football for your high school. If it doesn't hurt, it isn't good for you, right?

Wrong. Exercise works most of its miracles before pain even gets warmed up. You in fact do yourself a *disservice* by breaking into what physiologists call

---

Better to Slack Off Than Lay Off

We all have them: those periods when our exercise routines are pushed aside. Either we incur an injury, or we get "too busy," or we simply go through one of those spells when we tire of the obligation. It's natural. But it needn't be disastrous because, compared to getting in shape, staying in shape is easy. Only about half the effort required to achieve a level of fitness, in fact, appears to be enough to *maintain* that level.

Back in 1973, an experiment was done at Springfield College in Massachusetts in which "detraining" effects were studied. A group of people, after exercising 30 minutes a day five days a week for five weeks, were made to slack off to either four, three, two, or one session per week. Tested after five weeks on these reduced schedules, the people exercising four and three times a week had maintained virtually *all* of what their five-day-a-week schedules had gained them, and the twice-a-week and once-a-week groups came fairly close.

Moral of the story?

That you all-or-nothing types are doing yourself a disservice. If you're going to lay off, at least don't roll over and play dead. In just five weeks to two months, total inactivity can cost you everything you've worked for. But exercising even just once a week can retard the decline substantially. What's more, by punctuating your layoffs with even minimal activity, you avoid the "I've been off this long; what's one more day?" syndrome. And we all know how dangerous that can be.

As the researchers in charge of the experiment put it, "the fitness enthusiast who suddenly finds it difficult to exercise at his or her usual frequency due to business or other conflicts should consider a planned reduction in exercise frequency rather than stopping completely." Once cardiovascular fitness is acquired, it can be retained for an appreciable time by exercising less often (*Medicine and Science in Sports and Exercise*, vol. 5, no. 1, 1973).

anaerobic (not enough oxygen) metabolism too early in a workout. To improve the ability of the muscles to use oxygen, you've got to give them the amount they need—which, by getting out of breath, you do not do. Winding yourself early in an exercise session starves the muscles of oxygen, so they quit before they get a chance to get the workout they need.

"Train, don't strain." It's a rule that's been used by the world's top distance runners for years. And to it, we'd like to add another: "Don't do anything today that you wouldn't want to do again tomorrow." Life's too short.

E. Regular and Loving

The less we say to you people, the better. You've evidently cozied up to exercise in just the right way. Whatever you're doing, keep it up.

F. Compulsive

Whatever *you* people are doing, knock it off—just for a day. You will not turn into a pumpkin, and you will not get fat either.

What you *will* do is show yourself you have the confidence to do without. And a little bit of independence—in *any* relationship—is important.

The key to durability is flexibility. Keep that in mind the next time you go to suit up to run in the dark, with a cold, on a bad knee, in the rain.

26/

The Best Exercise Advice I Know

Have you ever wondered what the difference is between a fit muscle and an unfit one? It's a little like the difference between a small car engine and a big one: A big car engine usually has more spark plugs.

Inside of muscle tissue are tiny sites of energy production called mitochondria, which convert the food we eat into muscular activity (somewhat like spark plugs convert fuel into energy). The more we exercise, the more efficient —and more numerous—these little energy producers become. A well-conditioned muscle, in fact, can have as much as 50 percent more mitochondria than an unconditioned muscle. Which is why well-conditioned athletes can get away with eating so much: Not only are their muscles better at burning calories when they're exercising, but their muscles are also better at burning calories when they're at rest. Mitochondria, you see, have voracious appetites whether they're being used or not.

But in addition to being like spark plugs, mitochondria are also like tomatoes: Only so many can be grown in one spot. So the secret to having as many as possible is to plant them wherever you can—not just in the legs, as runners do, but all over. By working all muscles of the body, you saturate them all with mitochondria, and you wind up a much better calorie-burning machine as a result. Case in point: me.

I once checked out a fitness testing center which offered an underwater weighing test to determine percent body fat. And even though I run (only?) about 30 miles a week, I recorded the lowest percent body fat (4 percent) the center had encountered—about nine percent less, in fact, than most other runners tested.

Why?

Because I eat a low-fat, high-fiber diet, for one thing. But also because I exercise my upper half. And so my whole body—not just my legs—must be jam-packed with mitochondria just waiting to snatch up any calories they can get their hands on.

Man stays lean not by using his legs alone. To really wage war against fat, it's best to encourage the growth of mitochondria in as many "plots" as possible.

If you run, cycle, or walk, keep it up. The legs *are* your largest muscle group, and so exercise that involves them is great for burning calories. But if you really want to be an incinerator, you've also got to exercise your muscles from the waist up. Infiltrate these with mitochondria and you give fat a choice between a rock and a hard place.

What kind of upper body exercise is good?

Circuit weight training seems to be about the best because it's both strenuous and repetitive enough to work the heart and lungs. That seems to be the secret with mitochondria: They grow best in the presence of oxygen, and exercise that makes you huff and puff provides it. So if you're going to lift weights, choose fairly light ones, and do lots of "reps" rather than killing yourself on the heavy stuff. If you don't have access to weights, do chin-ups and push-ups. And cheat if you have to, in the beginning, by doing push-ups from your knees rather than toes, and by using a chair to help you get your chin up over that bar. The important thing is to get the muscles of your arms, chest, and back to burn calories in a way that gets you breathing. Because that's what builds mitochondria best.

Total body fitness. It's time has come. Not only can it keep you lean and mean, it can also keep you free of injury. By alternating workouts between upper body and lower, you give muscle groups the time they need to recuperate. Indeed, studies show that runners who work out three days a week have far fewer injuries than those who work out five or more.

So do your physique a favor: Give a little more time to your upper half.

Look Before You Leap into a Health Club

The fitness boom has created as much merchandise as it has muscle. We've now got everything from hand-held pulse monitors to jog-along radios. Which is fine. Motivation comes in different forms for different people. And for millions, that motivation has been in the form of the guidance and camaraderie that comes with joining a health club.

Should you join one?

That depends on you. If you're the type who needs structure and companionship, give one a try. Realize one thing, however: Unless you're prepared to invest effort as well as money, the only thing a health club is going to reduce is your bank account.

"Any club that says you can get in shape effortlessly is not telling you the truth," says Ruth Lindsey, Ph.D., professor of physical education at California State University at Long Beach. Dr. Lindsey has been checking out health club facilities since 1971, and has found more than a few to be frauds.

At many of these places, instructors get hired "mostly for their good looks," Dr. Lindsey said. They have no background in physical education; and, as a result, they often wind up misinforming patrons about the effects of exercise.

How can you smell out one of these "all show, no go" places before being asked to sign up? By doing some detective work, says former U.S. Olympic team physician Robert H. Pike, M.D. Take the time to "ask around about a club to see if there have been many dropouts," Dr. Pike advises. Then actually "sit down and talk with the club's manager, and interview some of its instructors." If they seem to know what they're talking about, then tour their facilities and see what they have to offer. If it's not a heck of a lot more than you have at home, look elsewhere.

Charles T. Kuntzleman, Ed.D., and the editors of *Consumer Guide*, in their book *Rating the Exercises* (William Morrow, 1978), recommend looking for a club that emphasizes cardiovascular fitness (the kind that increases the efficiency of the circulatory system by exercising the heart and lungs continuously for at least 20 minutes).

Dr. Lindsey agrees. "Look for a place that has facilities for exercises like jogging, swimming, and pedaling stationary bicycles," she says. "A strong heart is a matter of life and death." A bulging bicep is not.

Which brings us to the often controversial question of barbells. "If a club is set up to coach you properly, weight training and body building can be a valuable part of an exercise program," Dr. Pike feels. The best—and safest—strength-building equipment works on a principle of variable resistance by way of ropes, chains, and pulleys. (Nautilus and Universal Gym are two reputable names to look for.) The secret with weight training, as with any exercise program, Dr. Pike says, is to start out easy. Properly approached, it can tone and shape parts of your body that your cardiovascular program may not.

Do not, however, be dazzled by any chrome-plated gadgetry that purports to do your work for you. Passive exercise equipment (such as roller machines and belt vibrators) just plain don't work. As for the belt vibrators, "all they do," says Gabe Mirkin, M.D., in *The Sportsmedicine Book* (Little, Brown, 1978), "is shake your bladder and give you a headache."

Are saunas and steam rooms worth their price of admission?

For relaxing, maybe, but not for losing weight. In a sauna, the temperature of the air is high but its humidity is relatively low; in a steam room, things are both hot and wet. Neither can melt away fat the way exercise does.

Ward Dean, M.D., a naval flight surgeon, is one of the few people who believes there are any weight-reducing benefits to sweating at all. According to his calculations, your body expends about 0.6 calorie of energy for every gram of water it sweats. So after 10 to 15 minutes in a steam room or sauna, he says, you tax your cooling system to the tune of 100 to 200 calories, depending on how actively you ooze. (Be careful about stepping into a hot steam room or sauna after a hard workout, however. It's easier on your heart to get steamed up before you exhaust yourself.)

A health club, in other words, is what you make it. But it helps to have the right facilities to work with. As a precaution, check to see whether the club you're thinking of joining belongs to the Association of Physical Fitness Centers. The group is a trade association for full-service health spas and is dedicated to upgrading the industry.

Feel Good, Not Bad, about Missing a Workout

We all have them: those times when, for some reason, we just plain don't feel like working out. Not that we're ailing physically—it's a mental thing. We know our workouts are good for us. And we know they always make us feel better when we're done. And yet there are those times when we just feel like saying, "The heck with it."

So what do we do? Usually, one of two things.

We either do say, "The heck with it," which leaves us feeling guilty in addition to feeling grumpy.

Or we go ahead with the workout, which leaves us feeling resentful. Not right away, perhaps, but as our rosy glow wears off, resentment can emerge because it is human nature to resent anything that has power over us. And by exercising when we really don't want to, we are, in a sense, being coerced. I see two possible solutions to the problem.

One is to get to the bottom of why we get the urge to skip; the other is to arrive at a compromise which circumvents the skip. I'll explain the "why" approach first.

If the urge to miss comes over you often, your routine is either too difficult or too boring. And if difficulty is the problem, easing up is the solution. Better four easy workouts a week than two depressingly hard ones.

If boredom, on the other hand, is what's bugging you, try switching to a new routine. There is nothing inherently sacred about your present one, even if it has been with you for the past 15 years. And if burning your customary amount of calories is what you're worried about, keep in mind that the body begins to burn fewer calories as it gets progressively better at any given exercise. So by switching to something new—and being a little awkward at it—you stand to burn more calories than you would by waltzing through your routine of old.

If your reluctance to work out happens only very rarely, though, a change in routine may not be the answer. Maybe what's discouraging you is simply that there is something more important you feel you should be doing. That's happened to me. I get behind in my work and suddenly it feels as though I'm having to steal the time to exercise. The solution, I've found, is to get caught up in my work.

Or maybe it's simply a case of having something you'd rather do than work out. Nothing wrong with that.

It's important, in other words, to learn to show a little bit of respect for that antiexercise voice of yours, even if it does sometimes speak to you in a rebellious way. Because when part of you says it doesn't want to do something, it usually has a reason, however obscure that reason might be. And by always feeling compelled to keep your scheduled appointments with exercise, you risk labeling it a tyrant that you may eventually decide to overthrow for good.

Enough psychology. There's also a compromise approach you can take.

If you're not in a mood to work out, but you know that a little bit of exercise would make you feel better, then do just that: a little bit of exercise.

I've mastered the mini-workout quite well, if I do say so myself. I'll do some sit-ups, some jumping jacks, maybe some push-ups—just enough to break a sweat and feel as though I've earned a shower. (What is it about walking around with wet hair that can make you feel you've done something monumentally healthy?)

Or if calisthenics aren't your style, go for a walk, or a short bike ride, or a quick set of tennis. The mini-workout accomplishes two things: It revives you nearly as well as "the real thing," and it fends off the feeling of guilt associated with an out-and-out "miss."

How does it compare physiologically to your full-fledged workout?

That depends on your full-fledged workout. If you're doing enough in a mini-workout to get yourself breathing fairly heavily for 15 minutes or longer, you're at least not *losing* any fitness. Unless, of course, you're a world-class marathoner.

Exercise, in other words, need not be an all-or-nothing affair. And the sooner we all-or-nothing types realize that, the better. We would do better in the long run, in fact, to look at exercise as being like money in the bank: Every little bit counts.

It's interesting to note that when the running boom first started to make noise, runners would rate the worthiness of their training schedules in terms of daily mileage. Soon it became clear, though, that weekly totals were a more realistic way of keeping track. Now the thought is that monthly, perhaps even yearly, increments are the most realistic and meaningful way to evaluate accomplishment.

The point is: A miss here and there isn't going to hurt; it's long-term commitment that counts. And a certain degree of flexibility is very important in keeping long-term commitment alive.

So miss if you must—and don't worry about it.

And minimize if you can. And feel good about it.

As one of the world's greatest runners, Bill Rodgers, once told me, "I've learned to look at missed workouts as being able to help more than hurt me."

Wise words. We live with enough stress as it is. We don't need our exercise programs to burden us even more.

How to Run Two Miles in a Motel Room

It's one of those trips you can't stand: too long to avoid the overnight stay, too short to bother booking truly "accommodating" accommodations. Needing to clear your head after a less than perfect flight, you ask the desk clerk about the exercise facilities.

"The what?"

You kick yourself for not packing your running shoes, and return to your room . . . and to a T.V. that blinks.

Do not at this point head for the cocktail lounge. You can get a very good workout in motel a room.

Jumping jacks, sit-ups, push-ups, even chin-ups are possible (if the bar you hung your coat on is willing, and you don't mind bending your knees).

Start with jumping jacks. Five hundred may sound like a lot, but if you're in shape enough to be longing for a workout, you'll be through those 500 in about eight minutes, having burned about 100 calories (as many as you do jogging a mile) in the process. Because jumping jacks require you to spread your legs in a way that running does not, 500 of them could leave you a little sore. If you don't want to risk that, run in place for part of those eight minutes.

Caloric Costs of Selected Calisthenics

	Rate of Exercise (completed sequences per minute)	Energy Cost (calories)
Burpees (4-count)	14	9.3
Push-ups	28	6.5
Sprinter's stretch	14	4.7
Sit-ups, hands behind head	20	4.0
Knee raises, supine position	14	3.3
Alternate leg raises, supine position	10	2.5
Alternate toe touch, sitting	14	1.4
Side bends	14	1.2

SOURCE: Adapted from *The Physical Fitness Encyclopedia*, by Charles T. Kuntzleman (Emmaus, Pa.: Rodale Press, 1971).

Next, some sit-ups. If you can manage to eke out 60 (at a rate of 20 per minute), chalk up 12 more calories.

Push-ups. A set of 30 (done in a minute) is worth seven calories.

Alternate these exercises, but keep moving. The idea is to keep your heart clicking along at about the same rate as you would jogging, cycling, swimming, walking, or whatever. (Side bends, toe touches, and/or some other light stretching can be a good way to catch your breath between exercises like push-ups or chin-ups that may leave you puffing harder than you're used to.)

If you can keep yourself bopping along nonstop for about 20 minutes, you've gotten yourself a workout that's at least the equivalent of a two-mile run —and in the process you've gotten to some muscle groups that jogging doesn't.

Who knows—bounce around enough and you might shake some sense into that T.V.

Win—Don't Lose—an Unfit Spouse

As if the institution of marriage weren't in sad enough shape, there is now evidence to suggest that our newfound love affair with fitness could be straining the beleaguered custom even more. A poll taken at the most recent New York City Marathon, for example, showed that the divorce rate among participants was 340 percent above our national average (*Runner*, September, 1980).

Granted, marathon runners are not known for spending a lot of time around the house, but they reflect a growing trend nonetheless—toward self-improvement at all costs. Even if those costs include a spouse.

"The pursuit of fitness can make profound changes in people," cautions noted psychiatrist and author Thaddeus Kostrubala, M.D. Usually those changes are for the good, of course. But anytime something is good for one member of a relationship without being good for the other, it is apt to be bad for both, particularly now that we're striving to make marriage a pairing of equals.

We talked by phone with Dr. Kostrubala, and he assured us that the domestic dangers of fitness are very real. A veteran of 27 marathons and three marriages himself, the doctor said that the pursuit of fitness can be a symptom as well as a cause of marital strife. A husband who's running to get away from his wife, in other words, only makes things worse when he gets back.

Why should that be?

Because in a sense he's cheating. He's finding physical pleasure in something other than his wife's embrace. And a wife who exercises without her husband does the same. A strong element of jealousy can develop in a marriage where one member is fit and the other is not—a jealousy that easily can lead to resentment and worse.

We asked Dr. Kostrubala what might be done about minimizing those ill feelings between fit and unfit partners in a marriage, and he agreed with us that at the heart of reconciliation must be two things: a willingness to understand and a willingness to give.

It's time we, the fit, stopped just taking from our fitness programs and started sharing what we've gained. And if we can't do that, maybe what we've gained hasn't been worth the effort.

Enough philosophy: time for nuts and bolts. If you honestly think your spouse would be a healthier—and happier—person for being more fit, come up with some honest and imaginative encouragement. Not exhortation . . . encouragement. Because if there's anything that irks the unfit about the fit, it's an attitude of holier than thou. A few suggestions:

- If you run, invite your spouse to bike along. Or suggest trying a new sport together. Clumsiness likes company.
- Look for unique fitness programs being offered at spas or local Y's. And present what you find tactfully.
- Talk honestly about what fitness has done for you—honestly enough to admit its potential for becoming a negative, as well as a positive, addiction. Humility invites emulation.

And what if your humble encouragement fails?

That's when it's time for understanding. Because as much as it might sound like heresy for us to say it, exercise is not for everybody. There are some people for whom a regimented fitness program is simply too great a source of emotional or physical stress to be justified as a method for improving health. And the sooner we Jumping Jacks realize that, the better.

We must be careful not to let the self-fulfilling effects of our fitness efforts cloud our understanding of the needs of others. If and when the pursuit of fitness means the abandonment of compassion, I for one am all for abandoning fitness.

Stop Being Bored by Exercise

If fitness has a number one enemy, it isn't pain or inconvenience; it's boredom. I hear it all the time: "But doesn't all that exercise get boring?"

Well, my answer to that is no. Because in my particular case, I'm usually in too much pain to be bored. But as for the kind of fitness program that I recommend, I simply answer those people by saying, "Boredom is the absence of imagination."

And it's true. If you can't come up with an acceptably novel way of expending a certain number of calories per day in a way that you know is good for you, then it's not exercise, but rather *you* that's boring.

Think about it. Do you choose not to eat because it's boring? No. You come up with sufficient variety to keep eating rather fun. And do you avoid drinking because it's boring? We all know the answer to that.

Exercise should be considered a staple, just as food and drink are, so it's up to you to make it palatable. Here are a few ideas on how to do just that.

- Don't perform the same routine two days in a row. If familiarity breeds contempt, it does so on the basis of boredom. I've been working hard lately at mixing up my routine between running, riding a stationary bicycle, lifting weights—and even taking an occasional day off.
- Think about the benefits. Fantasize if you have to. My high school wrestling coach (the guy who was always saying, "What the mind can conceive, the body can achieve.") had trimmed that advice for himself into a world-class, body-building physique. You, however, might want to focus on something a bit closer to home: a set of less adorable love handles, perhaps. Or even just the prospect of a guilt-free beer.
- Find something that doesn't feel like exercise. If you like contests, this probably means bumping heads with others like yourself in games such as tennis, squash, racquetball, and touch football. But if you're the type who prefers to avoid confrontation, the solitude of jogging, walking, or cycling is more your style.
- Either do or do not count while you exercise. Admittedly that sounds noncommittal, but for people who are "counting" types, it helps. And for people who are not, it hurts. You won't know which you are, though, until you try.
- Exercise at different times of the day. Many people resist exercise simply because they resist routine. So don't make it routine. Exercise in the morning one day, the afternoon or evening the next. A different setting, too, can keep exercise novel. Vary your running or cycling routes. Life's too short to jog only one path.
- Keep aware of your surroundings. It can be very easy—and very depressing—to get locked up in the purely physical sensations of exercise. So say hello to people. Notice what kind of trash they put out and how well they keep their lawns cut. You can learn a lot about your neighborhood, and people in general, by keeping your eyes and ears open.
- Excite yourself occasionally. For you jet-setters that means setting your jet toward something that's good for you: skiing the Alps, hiking the Himalayas. (My idea of a high time, I'm afraid, is running up a certain hill a mile from my home around sunset.)

Learn When to Exercise

When's the best time to exercise?
I get asked that question a lot, especially by people just starting out. And

having tried everything from 6:00 A.M. to midnight myself, my answer would have to be: Whenever you most feel like it.

And the people in the labs agree with me. Individual body rhythms, digestive cycles, energy levels, mood swings, work schedules, and favorite T.V. shows vary so much that it would be impossible to prescribe one best time for everybody. So we'll do the next best thing. We'll help you come up with that "best time" yourself by considering two very basic questions.

First, Do you enjoy exercising?

And second, How does exercise make you feel?

If exercise is a chore, you'd probably best get it over with in the morning so you don't have to worry about it all day. Except, of course, if you hate exercise so much that the idea of a morning workout would keep you in bed until noon. In that case, we'd have to guess that there's something wrong with your exercise. No routine should be a cause for nightmares—so ease up. And then see if you can bear waking up to it.

For those of you who actually look forward to exercise, though, it might be better to hold it off until later, when you get home from work, perhaps, and feel you've earned your "recess."

Consideration number two: how exercise makes you feel. Some people it relaxes, others it peps up. If exercise relaxes you, we'd suggest saving it for early evening, such as before dinner, instead of a cocktail (or at least as a way of earning one).

If you find that exercise gives you a lift, however, we're back to our morning prescription, or our lunch hour one. Exercise for many people provides a kind of second wind. Much better than eating, in fact. (A friend of mine used to have a problem—falling asleep at around two o'clock every day. When I got him off the businessman's specials and on a bicycle during his lunch break, he pepped up—and slimmed down—considerably.)

Now, for some combinations.

If exercise does pep you up—but you're still not crazy about it—how about taking it in small but frequent doses. Some jumping jacks and toe touches before your shower in the morning to get the eyes open; a short walk for lunch instead of a slumberizing steak sandwich; a leisurely bike ride when you get home from work to perk you up for a worthwhile evening. That's the way our prehistoric ancestors got their exercise: often and easy.

But if you're the type who likes to go hard and then rest up, that's okay, too. It doesn't matter so much how and when you put in the time, just so long as you put in the time. Two thousand calories' worth of exercise a week. According to a study done several years ago by Ralph S. Paffenbarger, M.D., D.P.H., of Stanford University, men who did that amount of exercise reduced their chances of heart disease substantially (*American Journal of Epidemiology*, September, 1978). The following table should help you make appropriate calculations.

Calories Used per Hour
of Selected Activities

	Activity Level	Weight (pounds)		
		125	170	220
Basketball	moderate	352	476	624
	vigorous	495	668	877
Bicycling	5.5 miles per hour, level	251	339	444
	13 miles per hour, level	537	726	952
Fencing	moderate	251	339	444
	vigorous	513	693	909
Golf	twosome	271	367	481
	foursome	203	275	361
Handball	vigorous	488	660	866
Rowing, machine or scull	20 strokes per minute	684	924	1,212
Running	5.5 miles per hour, level	537	726	952
	7 miles per hour, level	699	945	1,239
	9 miles per hour, level	777	1,050	1,378
	2.5 percent grade	907	1,225	1,607
	4 percent grade	959	1,295	1,699
	12 miles per hour	984	1,330	1,744
	in place (140 counts per minute)	1,222	1,650	2,164
Soccer		447	604	793
Squash		520	703	922
Tennis	moderate	347	468	614
	vigorous	488	660	866

SOURCE: Fitness Finders, Inc., 1969.

There are, however, some times when exercise is *not* advisable:

- *directly after a large meal.* Wait at least two hours. Digestion requires a substantial amount of blood flow to the stomach. And when you're exercising, your muscles are going to be wanting that blood. What's more, a feeling of fullness can make breathing difficult, and nausea easy.
- *under the influence of alcohol.* Alcohol is a strange fuel. It supplies calories (6.2 per gram) but those calories, unfortunately, are such that they demand more oxygen for metabolization than you (if you're exercising) are in a position to spare. The result is apt to be weakness and, depending on the amount consumed, lack of coordination and good sense.

- *when you're injured or when you're ill.* That may sound obvious to some of you, but to you exercise addicts, it may sound intimidating. The human body is not a metronome; it needs occasional intermissions to keep the beat going on.

Get Workouts with Your Kids

If you've got any children around the house between the ages of about 4 and 20, for fitness' sake don't waste them: Do your best to keep up with them and you'll be doing everybody a favor.

The notion of "aerobic parenthood" occurred to me one night. I had, for one reason or another, missed my morning run, and having gotten home too late that evening to run before dark, I was contemplating mixing myself a stiff drink as an act of surrender when my four-year-old daughter started telling me about what a great time she and Mom had had at the playground that day.

"Think *you* could take me sometime, Dad?"

"Sure, Elizabeth. Maybe next weekend."

"They keep the lights on until 8:00," came my wife's voice from the kitchen.

Well, we went. And I'll be darned if I didn't get my workout after all. Fourteen times up (and down) the sliding board; 15 breathtaking minutes on the swings; *twice* across the monkey bars (I was stiff for three days); and finally, a grueling ten minutes of deep knee bends on the seesaw. (Elizabeth weighs only 42 pounds.)

Maybe you've got a stringy nine-year-old who needs work on ground balls. Or a teenager with a weak backhand. Get to work on them. It's a great way to supplement whatever else you're doing to keep in shape. But more than that, it's a great way to keep *them* in shape. Laboratory experiments have shown that rats are less apt to become obese later in life if they are made to exercise during their periods of growth. Reporting in *Physiology of Exercise* (William C. Brown, 1980), Herbert A. deVries, Ph.D., of the University of Southern California, says, "To the extent that these data may be extrapolated to the human, it would seem possible to prevent the laying down of excess numbers of adipose [fat] cells by providing adequate physical activity for young children and adolescents. Physical activity," Dr. deVries says, "appears to be even more important than eating habits."

Drink Water When You're Thirsty

Beverage companies have been admirably energetic in trying to accommodate the thirsts of the fitness boom's perspiring millions. But they have also, unfortunately, been a bit wrong. Most of the ergogenic (performance-improving) beverages being produced commercially today are simply too rich. By offering electrolytes (minerals lost during sweating) and sugar in too concentrated a form, they slow the absorption of what you need most after strenuous exercise—water. For that reason, the American College of Sports Medicine (ACSM) recommends that if you do drink a commercially prepared athletic tonic, you at least do your thirst the favor of watering it down according to the accompanying guidelines.

Dilution Guidelines for Common Beverages

	Calories*	Carbo- hydrates* (grams)	Parts Water to Add
Energade	120	30	5
Gatorade	48	12	2
Quickick	44	11	2
Super Socco	125	31	5
Wagner Thirst	76	19	3
Apple juice	120	29.6	5
Grape juice	167	42	7
Orange juice	122	28.9	5
V-8 juice	47	10.6	2
Country Time Lemonade	90	22	4
Hawaiian Punch	120	30	5
Coca-Cola	96	24	4
Dr. Pepper	99	24.8	4
Seven-Up	96	24	4

NOTES: *Per eight ounces of beverage cited.
Because carbohydrate (glucose) concentrations greater than six grams per eight ounces can retard absorption, the American College of Sports Medicine recommends that the above beverages be diluted as shown.

SOURCE: Adapted from "Nutrition Update Fluid Replacement Beverages," by Patricia Beckwith (*Sportsmedicine Digest*, May, 1981).

"When glucose [alias sugar, represented by carbohydrate on the chart] is made available to an athlete during lengthy exercise, it should be provided in low concentrations," explains Edward L. Fox, Ph.D. (*Sports Physiology*, W. B. Saunders, 1979). "The stomach can empty only a limited amount of glucose in a short period of time; if too much glucose is present, the rate of gastric emptying is retarded."

Wolfing down a can of soda between sets, in other words, is apt to revive you less than a glass of plain water, because your body needs water more than sugar to perform in the heat. Sugar in the soda slows the rate at which the water in soda can be absorbed.

"A water loss of just 3 percent [that's six pounds—or six pints of sweat —if you're a 200-pounder] may significantly diminish exercise performance and provoke heat illness," warns Dr. Fox. For that reason he recommends "frequent water breaks (e.g., every 10 to 15 minutes)" to keep the body's water table from approaching that 3 percent deficit.

And as for those highly advertised electrolytes, we get enough of them (especially sodium) in the food we eat. Only under the most extreme circumstances (sweat losses of six pounds or more) can taking salt tablets be justified —and only then along with adequate amounts of water. "Taking salt tablets without adequate water is far worse than taking no salt tablets at all," cautions Dr. Fox. The recommended ratio is one pint of water for every seven-grain tablet taken.

And what about beer?

Considering one 12-ounce can contains about 13 grams of carbohydrate, 25 milligrams of sodium, and 90 milligrams of potassium, your favorite brew would pass the ACSM's recommendations—if you could stomach diluting it with 12 ounces of water. If it's beer you must have after a workout, you're better off with one of the "light" brews, which have carbohydrate contents (from one to six grams per 12 ounces) that come closer to what the ACSM recommends.

Still, though, the "real thing" when it comes to replacing body fluids is plain old water. "Water is the best and most easily available fluid replacement beverage for competition," states Patricia Beckwith, R.D., M.P.H., in *Sportsmedicine Digest* (May, 1981). You might want to keep that in mind the next time you're given the option of water or an electrolyte beverage during your next fun run.

Advice from Bill Rodgers

Several years ago, I had a chance to interview marathoner Bill Rodgers. Bill was in his prime then, so what he told me was of great significance indeed.

"To do well in this sport, you've really got to think—and be flexible. I used to get into arguments in college about what it meant to be intelligent. One classmate of mine, who must have weighed 350 pounds, was of the mind that it was all in the head. I'd always thought it was just as smart to take care of yourself physically—so you could be around as long as possible to enjoy yourself."

I liked the logic of that. But I couldn't help wondering how training to run 130 miles a week could be enjoyable.

"Oh, it's grueling sometimes. But I've decided this is going to be a very intense period of my life. It's a great thrill to win big races. And I'm going to do all I can right now to do it. But I'll tell you, I'm not going to be sorry when it comes time to put all this behind me. Because then I'll be able to go back to running the way I got started in the first place—for the sheer fun of it."

I asked Bill how far his "sheer fun" would be taking him as a retiree.

"Somewhere between 30 and 50 miles a week. My longest runs will be maybe 10 miles—on weekends, that kind of thing. And I'll probably ride a bike, and swim, and play tennis."

At that point in his career, Bill was running about 18 miles a day, usually in two separate workouts, at a pace between 6 and 6½ minutes per mile. I asked him how much he thought was enough for the rest of us, for the sake of general fitness.

"Two, maybe three miles every other day. The important thing is to be consistent. And to do that, it helps to like it. Which is why I've always said to people: 'Do whatever it is you enjoy.' Tennis, racquetball, swimming, walking, riding a bike. The only reason I run as much as I do is because of my focus on the marathon. I feel I've been blessed with a talent, and I want to make the most of it while I can."

Bill had not always been so dedicated to his ability. There were several years after college when he did not run at all. And, he smoked cigarettes . . .

"About a pack a day. And I was in the bars a lot, too. It wasn't a good period of my life. I was concerned about staying out of the draft. Running was the last thing on my mind."

So what gave a wayward dropout the sense of direction to become what many (including myself) consider to be one of the greatest marathoners of all time?

"I saw some people I had run against in college do pretty well in the Boston Marathon. And I got some encouragement from friends and my wife, Ellen. And so gradually I got back into it. And the more I ran, the more I realized I had a talent for running. It seemed to fit my personality. So I pushed it."

At that point I felt comfortable enough to ask Bill to do something my brother had dared me I wouldn't: to arm wrestle. He let out a laugh at my request, and went on humbly to announce that he had been beaten two weeks earlier by female marathoner Patti Lyons. I (5'9" and 145 pounds) promised to go easy on him (5'9", 128) as we cleared his desk . . .

Do not let the man's willow branch arms deceive you: There's a heart of an oak behind them. Having a set a chin-up record in college, I was more than a little shocked at how long it took me to beat him.

When I'd a chance to catch my breath (Bill never lost his), I confessed my surprise. He seemed flattered.

"I guess I am stronger than some runners, because I work out with weights. Mostly in the winter, though, when it's not so hot. In this kind of weather I'm just too whipped after a hard workout to put in the extra time at the gym."

Our tussle had relaxed things to the point where I felt I could ask Bill how a prerace training schedule of 170 miles a week (which he's now doing to get ready for New York) affected his sex drive. For the first time in our interview he hesitated.

"I guess I'd have to say that it makes me less apt to get involved. But when I do, the sex is better. I seem to have more energy."

We joked about the relevance of this to the bumper stickers about runners making better lovers and then moved on to the subject of diet. I told Bill he had a reputation for leaving good nutrition in the dust.

"That's not true. I have a very good diet. I might eat a few too many simple carbohydrates—cakes, cookies, candy, and that kind of thing—but otherwise I'm very careful about what I eat."

I asked for a rundown of a typical day's intake.

"Okay. Today, for example, I had a cup of coffee for breakfast, and a big salad and some peanut butter for lunch. Tonight I'll have another big salad and some turkey and maybe some ham. I was tested once, and they told me I was getting about four thousand calories a day."

Bill's diet seemed to parallel rather nicely his approach to life: health via happiness. I asked him to what degree alcohol now fit into that philosophy.

"Oh, I still drink. Mixed drinks mostly. I like gin and tonics. And rum. And beer. I guess I'll average maybe a drink a day. But I won't go out anymore and get zapped the way I used to. It's not worth it."

We should all be so wise.

SECTION III/REST

In a world that wants us out late and up early, the secret to getting adequate rest is to learn to find it in ways other than sleep.

27/

Stretching: The Difference
a Little Flexibility Can Make

"It isn't prime rib that causes heart attacks; it's the prime rate."

I made that remark to a friend of mine in the real estate business one night as we mulled over what to have for dinner at a posh restaurant, and for as little thought as I had put into it, it seemed—particularly to him—to make some sense. There are mental as well as physical causes for disease, we decided, and the worst offenders may be the mental ones that we can't control. So what do we do about them, if we can't control them?

I began telling my friend about experiments being done that show how physical exercise can make us "less brittle targets." He was not at that point an exerciser, so my lecture struck him about as I might have expected.

"What's exercise going to do—make me so tired I'm not going to give a damn?"

"If you were to overdo it, yes," I conceded.

"But just the right amount of exercise can merely refresh you to the point where you are not taking it personally every time the interest rate goes up a percentage point."

To make a long story short, I got my friend to begin his days with about 20 minutes of calisthenics and stretching, and "whether it's just in my head or what," he recently told me, "things don't seem to bother me quite so much anymore."

Well, it *was* in his head, I told him, but that was good because that's where "it" belonged. Exercise may involve the muscles, but it's felt by the brain. There's a physical side and a mental side to being able to relax, and what exercise does is put our bodies in a "mood" that our minds can more easily follow up on.

"In the last ten years, we have conducted five different studies in young, middle-aged, and older men and women in which appropriate exercise has been shown to improve the ability to relax both immediately and over a sustained period," writes Herbert A. deVries, Ph.D., in *Vigor Regained* (Prentice Hall, 1974). Dr. deVries is director of the Mobile Laboratory for Physiology of

Exercise and Aging Research at the University of Southern California. He likes to tell the story of a certain retired businessman for whom exercise proved particularly therapeutic.

He had spent his professional life as a jewelry manufacturer, and for years had been eating aspirin "like peanuts" for tension headaches, says Dr. deVries. When he started our program, tests disclosed that the electrical activity in his muscles was higher than average, indicating that he was tense and unable to relax as well as he might. After five months of physical conditioning, his muscular activity was down by 63 percent. And his headaches were gone.

In another experiment conducted by Dr. deVries, this one using highly anxious patients from a medical center in California, physical conditioning reduced electrical muscle activity by an average of 20 to 25 percent, while neither a single dose of a tranquilizer nor a placebo had any effect at all. The amount of exercise responsible for these results, moreover, was "the laboratory equivalent," Dr. deVries said, "of a brisk 15-minute walk."

How does exercise work its tranquilizing magic?

There are several explanations. Even just moderate exercise has the ability to raise the temperature of muscles enough to make them less tense. More vigorous exercise that is sustained for 30 minutes or more, however, has the ability to release actual painkilling (and mood-elevating) chemicals into the brain. Some scientists see this as an evolutionary holdover from the days when it was not uncommon for extended physical efforts to be necessary for survival. Our bodies, so the theory goes, learned to medicate themselves against the pain of such experiences—naturally.

But exercise isn't the whole story. It's very important to keep loose as you exercise. Flexibility is key, because joint mobility and muscular pliability allow nerve impulses to flow as they should, particularly as we get older. Many scientists believe that aging muscles, especially those deprived of exercise, undergo a shortening process. And as muscles shorten, they put pressure on the nerves that run through them. Hence, the aches and pains we associate with old age.

Many of these, however, are avoidable, Dr. deVries says. "The best way to insure against the physical discomforts that so often accompany the aging process is to maintain an optimum level of physical fitness with appropriate emphasis on improvement of joint mobility." And that means *stretching*. Not before, but rather *after* you exercise.

"Never stretch unless you are thoroughly warmed up," says Ben E. Benjamin, Ph.D., author of *Sports without Pain* (Summit Books, 1979). Cold muscles resist stretching, whereas muscles that are "warm and surging with blood" are pliable. Muscles are like honey, he says; the colder they are, the stiffer they are. Always do a minimum of 5 to 15 minutes of exercise to get them ready.

Got that? It runs counter to what you may have been told in high school or college. But then, sportsmedicine is a relatively new science—one which has learned, too, that there are *right* as well as *wrong* ways to go about the act of stretching itself. Make note of the following no-nos.

- *Never "bounce" when you stretch.* The familiar first lunge that people make when they go to touch their toes, for example, actually does more harm than good. It arouses what physiologists call the "splinting reflex," meaning muscles react to such abuse by contracting rather than lengthening. The idea is to *ease* into a stretch, slowly, and hold it as long as it is reasonably comfortable.
- *Don't try to stretch a muscle while it's bearing weight.* Your legs, for example. Stretching leg muscles in a standing position is not as effective as stretching them while sitting or lying down, because in a standing position your leg muscles are contracted.

Keeping those instructions in mind, take a look at the following stretches. We picked these (among hundreds of possibilities) because they focus on the muscles of the lower body and neck, those which are subject to the most tension during your working day. Do them daily, if you can. And after, rather than before, you've gotten yourself warm.

Back stretch.   Sitting on the floor with your legs straight and spread about a foot apart, lean forward in an attempt to put your head between your knees. You should feel a stretching sensation in the backs of your legs and the small of your back. You can pull yourself forward by holding on to your lower legs or toes, if you want. Try to hold a slightly painful position for several seconds before you let go.

Wall lean.   Place your hands against a wall at about shoulder height and begin to inch your feet slowly backwards, keeping your heels on the floor. When you get to a point where you feel a burning sensation in the backs of your calves, hold the position for about ten seconds, then move forward for relief. Repeat several times.

Neck stretch.   While either sitting or standing, clasp your hands behind your neck and let your head fall forward. Hold this position for 10 to 15 seconds, then raise your head and rest. You can move your hands higher up on your skull for a greater pull. But be careful—don't hurt yourself. Two or three times should be enough.

Stretch your imagination as well as your muscles. If you don't like these exercises, come up with some of your own. Anything that feels as though it's stretching a tight area of your body is fair game. And for those of you *really* interested in loosening up, look into yoga. It's the state of the art, and has some very practical applications despite its eccentric image.

28/

Sleep: It's the Quality,
Not the Quantity, That Counts

Winston Churchill functioned best on about five hours. But then Albert Einstein was a zombie on anything less than nine. "One of the most pervasive myths about sleep," says sleep expert Dr. Wilse B. Webb, "is that everybody needs eight hours."

Ernest Hartmann, M.D., director of the Tufts University School of Medicine Sleep Laboratory, agrees. "There are long sleepers and short sleepers," he says, "and people who fall in between." The name of the game when it comes to sleeping well is to determine which you are—and then not fight it.

Say, for example, you have a "big day" tomorrow, one for which you want to be at your very best. Should you go to bed early, expecting to wake up ready to lick the world?

Not unless you go to bed early every night, the experts say. Researchers at the Montefiore Hospital Sleep-Wake Disorders Center in New York City have discovered that going to bed early to ensure getting enough sleep can be a waste of time. Everybody has his own personal body clock which dictates when sleep—for optimum results—should be taken. It has to do with your body's metabolic rhythm, and to go against this rhythm can be counterproductive. Sleep, especially dreaming, is work for the brain. And by forcing more on yourself than you need, you can suffer some rather classic symptoms of overdose, such as grogginess and feelings of disorientation. With sleep, as with exercise, more is not necessarily better.

Consistency is the key to getting the most out of your hours in bed, experts agree. Your body functions best when put on a schedule, however out of the ordinary that schedule may seem.

Sleep, in other words, is like food: Everybody's needs are different. Due to factors which experts list as age, heredity, health, lifestyle, occupational stress, and, to a large degree, personality, there are as many versions of "a good night's sleep" as there are sleepers.

Experts, for the sake of science, however, like to fit us into either of two very general groups.

Short sleepers, they say, tend to be dynamos, people of action who are 141 energetic, ambitious, and eager to excel within the standards of society. They waste little time worrying, and when problems do plague them, they lose themselves in their work. Many successful politicians, businessmen, and career soldiers make up the ranks of short sleepers.

Long sleepers, on the other hand (good for anything over 8½ hours), are apt to be writers, artists, and philosophers—people who use their sleep (dream sleep especially) to mull over and splice new ideas into their minds.

Whichever type of sleeper you are, though, it's important to make your hours in bed productive ones. From all the current research data available, we have compiled the following tips to help you do that.

- Try to get your sleep at the same time every night. Ben Franklin with his "early to bed and early to rise" was right, but only in the sense that what's important is sticking to a schedule.
- Make certain—through experimentation—that the hours you *are* sleeping are good ones. This can be done by keeping a sleep log (see accompanying box).
- Exercise—but not before bed. Your body needs a good two hours, sometimes more, to cool down after a workout.
- Don't get your mind racing before bed by working on something important. Your brain, like your body, needs time to cool off.
- Steer clear of sleeping pills and alcoholic nightcaps. The sleep promoted by these artificial aids is not the real thing.
- Try to get into a relaxing bedtime ritual. A set routine can set up patterns that suggest sleep to your mind just as convincingly as sticking to fixed hours suggests sleep to your body.
- Keep cool. Studies have shown that people sleep best at temperatures *under* 70°F.
- Have sex, but only if you find it relaxing. If it tends to invigorate you, save it for the morning.
- Make sure you have a comfortable bed.
- Don't go to bed hungry. Sometimes a drop in blood sugar during the night (not to mention a growling stomach upon retiring) can interfere with sleep. Eating the right foods, however, can prevent that.

In fact, this last point may be the most important. Scientists have found that a judicious mixture of before-bed foods may be your best ticket to dreamland. Protein-rich foods, for instance, contain an amino acid called tryptophan which has been proven an effective sleep inducer in a number of laboratory experiments. The substance works by reducing levels of chemicals in the brain (catecholamines) that tend to keep us awake.

Alice Kuhn Schwartz, Ph.D., coauthor of the book *Somniquest* (Harmony, 1979), explains that to get enough tryptophan we have to monitor not only the *what* we eat but also *when*.

"Animal studies have shown that eating carbohydrate foods—those that are starchy or sweet—liberates tryptophan and gives it greater access to the brain. In fact, the tryptophan in food is hardly used at all by the brain unless a carbohydrate food is also eaten.

"The implications of this are fascinating," she says. "If you've been eating high-protein, high-tryptophan foods during the day, and you want to fall asleep at night, then it may help to eat some bread, have a banana, drink some grape

---

Improve Your Sleep: Keep a Sleep Log

Could a few bad habits be interfering with your sleep more than you realize? One way to find out is to keep a sleep log—a daily record of the circumstances under which you approach your nightly rest. For a period of two weeks, keep track of:

- the time you go to bed.
- the time you wake up.
- how long you think it takes you to fall asleep.
- the total time you sleep.
- how you feel each morning when you awake.

For each of these 14 nights, also note:

- what you have to eat or drink, or what medications you take.
- what you do each evening before going to bed (read, work, watch T.V., socialize, or whatever).
- what you do each *day* in the way of exercise.
- how much coffee, tea, hot chocolate, or cola you have from noon on.
- whether or not you give in to napping at any time during the day.

At the end of the two weeks, sit down and compare the bad nights' sleep with the circumstances of the days both preceding *and* following them. It's likely you'll see some patterns develop. Zero in on the circumstances surrounding those restless nights—and learn from them.

By making habits of more of the conditions that seem to associate *positively* with sleep (and less of those that associate *negatively* with it), you should be able to improve the quality of your sleep substantially.

or apple juice, or have some figs or dates—all high-carbohydrate foods that can help activate tryptophan." But . . .

If your problem with sleep is that it takes you a while to get there, it's important that you do your carbo-snacking two to four hours before tucking in to give the appropriate chemical reactions the time they need to take effect.

If, on the other hand, your trouble is not so much falling asleep as staying there, then you should do your snacking immediately before retiring, thus insuring that your dietary nightcap begins to feel snug when *you* need it most.

And what if you wake up in the middle of the night with a lean and hungry look?

It's too late to do much about it then, Dr. Schwartz says. What's more, "there's a small child in all of us that will get used to waking up every night expecting to be rewarded . . . and it will become a habit." You're better off getting up and doing something extremely boring for those occasional late-night awakenings, Dr. Schwartz says.

The formula, then, is this: Carbohydrates eaten either *with* or several hours *after* protein foods equals increased tryptophan availability to the brain, and hence drowsiness.

For your tryptophan sources, look to the protein foods listed in the table. We've noted their tryptophan contents in milligrams per 100-gram (3½-ounce) portions. As for the carbohydrate segment of your sleep treat, fresh fruits, fruit juices, whole grain breads, cereals, and yes, even cookies (if you must) are fair game.

Foods That Can Help You Sleep

	Tryptophan* (milligrams)	Calories*
Cheddar cheese	341	398
Peanuts, roasted	340	585
Turkey, light meat, roasted	340	176
Tuna, canned in oil, drained	285	197
Tuna, canned in water	277	127
Chicken, roasted	250	290
Beef, chuck	217	327
Cottage cheese, 4 percent fat	179	106
Milk, skim	49	36
Milk, whole	49	65
Yogurt	20	61

NOTE: *Per 100 grams of food cited.

SOURCES: U.S. Department of Agriculture Handbook nos. 8, 8–1, and 8–5; and *Amino Acid Contents of Food*, Home Economic Report no. 4, by Martha Louise Orr and Bernice K. Watt (Washington, D.C.: Agricultural Research Service, U.S. Department of Agriculture, 1968).

29/
Transcendental Meditation: Something to Think About

I know Rick Levy well enough to have joked with him about something dear to his heart: "Transcendental meditation—that's learning to mumble in your sleep, right?"

Rick, who's been a certified TM instructor for nearly seven years now, smiled a little uneasily, not sure whether I was really expecting an answer.

I was, though. In my own clumsy way.

Rick and I have known each other on and off since about 1970, but his affiliation with TM had always confused me. Because not only is Rick a twice-a-day meditator, he's also a five-to-eight-mile-a-day runner, an executive in the clothing manufacturing business, an accomplished songwriter, and a dedicated father. Somehow Rick's earthly endeavors have never quite jived with my image of meditators as people on the lookout for cloud nine. We decided to iron out my confusions about TM in a "formal" interview at my place after a Sunday morning run.

P.S.: Why run *and* meditate? Don't the two do the same thing—relax you?

R.L.: Yes, but not in quite the same way. Running is relaxing and beneficial in a physical sense, whereas TM—transcendental meditation—is relaxing and beneficial more in a mental way.

P.S.: How do you mean beneficial?

R.L.: Meditation, I guess you could say, does for the mind what exercise does for the body. It gets it in shape.

P.S.: Wait a minute. Push-ups for the brain?

R.L.: In a sense. There seems to be a change in brain activity during TM, and that produces a greater mental clarity in everyday life. What I've noticed in my own life is that I've become much better able to remain objective about things. And I think I'm a lot more resilient to stress. 145

P.S.: How do you know it hasn't been your running that's done that for you?

R.L.: Oh, I'm sure my running has helped. But I was a meditator before I was a runner. I think meditation helped me become a runner.

P.S.: And a songwriter, and all the rest?

R.L.: All I can say is that I'm doing a lot more now than I ever thought I would.

P.S.: Can anybody learn to meditate?

R.L.: Anybody who can think can meditate. We've taught five-year-old kids TM. It's a much simpler and more mechanical process than many people realize.

P.S.: Where does the mantra fit in, and what is it exactly?

R.L.: It's just a meaningless sound which the instructor has been taught how to pick to suit you, as an individual. There is nothing mystical or magical about it.

P.S.: Do you get many people who can't "get into" it?

R.L.: Some people stop after a while, probably because they're trying to achieve a peaceful state of mind during TM. The technique is so effortless, and people in our society are so used to achieving results, that a person can begin to meditate incorrectly, stop feeling benefits in his daily life, and so give up the practice. But we TM teachers provide "checking" to make sure a person is meditating correctly, and I've never known anyone to stop who was being checked regularly.

P.S.: You meditate twice a day for 20 minutes. Isn't that hard to fit into your day?

R.L.: Not really. I meditate in the morning when I get up. And then again when I get home before dinner. I've known executives to meditate on trains, planes.

P.S.: So you're not asleep when you meditate, then.

R.L.: No. You're in a state deeper than sleep. But you're conscious.

P.S.: Conscious enough not to miss your stop?

R.L.: Sure.

P.S.: Does it leave you feeling refreshed?

R.L.: Usually it does—especially if I'm feeling tired going into a session. Then it leaves me noticeably revitalized.

P.S.: Do you see a change in yourself right away?

R.L.: No. It's very subtle, which in the beginning may turn a lot of people off. But running doesn't make any great noticeable changes right away, either. Both take time. Normally people begin to notice things within a month to six weeks.

P.S.: Sounds good, Rick. But does it really work?

R.L.: Well, there are over a million people who practice TM in America. And over two million throughout the world. I know it's worked for me, and I guess it's working for them.

Rick was nice enough not to kick me when I ended our interview by falling off my chair muttering, "Ommm. . . ."

30/
Music: A Way of Altering Your Mood without Altering Your Health

On one level, you've got a teenager barreling down Main Street mesmerized by the carnal roar of the Rolling Stones.

On another, you've got cancer patients being soothed by the flowing harmonies of Debussy.

Music is powerful stuff.

Healers in ancient times used music to treat heart problems, to lift depression, and to cure insomnia. It worked as medicine then. And it can work even better today. Because today there is more noise for music to drown out.

Ernest A. Peterson, Ph.D., chief of the Division of Auditory Research at the University of Miami School of Medicine, did an experiment which suggests that the amount of noise we live with today could be doing us harm.

Dr. Peterson took a healthy rhesus monkey and for one day exposed it to normal levels of everyday twentieth-century noise. The ring of an alarm clock, the buzz of an electric razor, and the dialogue of the "Today Show" made up the first part of the monkey's morning. Following 30 minutes of canned traffic, it was on to a nine-to-five symphony of workday racket. Nightfall brought televised football. And the monkey's sleep, finally, was lightly polluted by the hum of a room air conditioner.

How did he hold up?

Not well. His blood pressure and heart rate increased 30 percent, and stayed elevated long after relative peace was restored. "These results are not definitive," Dr. Peterson remarked on the findings, "but they do suggest to us that noise may be one of the factors contributing to the long-term development of cardiovascular disease in man."

Why is noise so upsetting?

Because we're still not used to it. While technological progress has brought with it a veritable holocaust of sound, we remain stuck inside bodies that evolved during times of relative quiet. Big noises for the caveman meant big trouble, be it in the form of an approaching lion or a volcanic eruption. Our bodies haven't quite been able to forget that.

148

We may *think* we've adapted to the clamor of the twentieth century, says Jack Westman, M.D., professor of psychiatry at the University of Wisconsin, Madison. But subconsciously, it's weighing on us, he says.

When a group of 960 housewives were interviewed in Denmark, for example, it was found that those who lived in loud neighborhoods (with noise levels in the 69 to 78 decibel range) saw doctors more often for psychological problems, used more tranquilizers, and showed higher rates of mental illness than women living in areas where decibel levels were between 51 and 63.

Noise has a way of "bringing to the surface submerged tensions," Dr. Westman says. He sees it as a catalyst to more warfare along the domestic front than many of us realize.

So what do we do about noise if—as Dr. Westman says—there is no healthy way of simply tuning it out?

We can do our best to eliminate it. Or we can reverse its disquieting effects by exposing ourselves to its opposite: music.

If noise is sound out of order, music is sound *in* order. And the more ordered this sound is, the better it is for us.

An interesting example of this comes from a study done in West Germany which showed that professional musicians, while rehearsing discordantly modern compositions (made up of "arbitrary sounds and noises"), complained of nervous tension, headaches, depression, difficulty sleeping, marital and family problems, and even impotence—*none* of which were a problem when these musicians rehearsed classical scores. Flatly stated by the *German Tribune*, "The majority of these musicians are convinced that their health is suffering from constant recitals of contemporary music."

"Music," in other words, can do damage as well as good. It is, indeed, powerful stuff.

How does it work?

Along two fronts, basically. Music has rhythm, a "beat" which works on us physically. And it has a melody, a "tune" which works on us psychologically.

For example, John Diamond, M.D., former professor of psychiatry at Mount Sinai Hospital in New York, did an experiment which showed that when people listened to a drumbeat characteristic of much of today's rock and roll, they were robbed of two-thirds of their muscular strength. Because the beat (two shorts followed by a long) is the exact inverse of the rhythm of the heart, it interferes with the transmission of brain waves from one side of the brain to the other, Dr. Diamond says, and the result is muscular weakness. The beat of a waltz, on the other hand (*one*, two, three; *one*, two, three), had a strengthening effect, he determined.

What can melody do? Put the finishing touches on rhythm. What rhythm starts (physically), melody finishes (emotionally). In a work of art, the two cooperate, and the result can be a very moving experience.

So what can all that mean for you?

A way to "alter your consciousness" without having to alter your health.

The next time you find yourself in a mood that you either (*a*) don't like or (*b*) wouldn't mind amplifying, try putting on some music.

If your mood is low, don't rush it. Start out with something even sadder than you are, to "bleed" yourself. Then work up gradually to happier pieces.

By the same token, if you're wound up, and would like to wind down, try irritating yourself that final "inch" with something just as hyper as you are. *Then* work down to where you want to be. Don't make the mistake of trying to do too much, too fast. Establish a rapport first between yourself and music. Then start taking "trips."

If all this sounds like so much hippie hogwash, we're sorry. But we'll bet you three songs on the jukebox that, given a chance, music could add some very worthwhile accents to your life.

When to Listen to What

Making specific recommendations is difficult, because music relies on personal associations for a large part of its effect. We'll try, nevertheless.

To relax. Look to lightly orchestrated pieces with easy rhythmic flow: Debussy's "Clair de lune," Wagner's "Song to the Evening Star" from *Tännhauser*, Dvorak's "New World Symphony."

To perk up. Try selections with pronounced and bouncy rhythms: Gounod's "Soldier Chorus," Berlioz's "Hungarian March," Gershwin's "Rhapsody in Blue," Sousa's "Stars and Stripes Forever."

To fall asleep. Some good ones are "The Slumber Motif" from Wagner's *Die Walküre*, Strauss's "Blue Danube," "The Bartered Bride" by Bach.

To lift your spirits. Try Chopin's mazurkas and preludes, Schubert's "Faith in Spring," the melodious arias of Verdi and Bellini, Mozart's sonatas, the first and second movements of Beethoven's Fourth Symphony, or the slower movement of Beethoven's Eighth.

Put these pieces on—or others like them—as background music, or give them your undivided attention. The nice thing about music is that it works whether you concentrate on it or not. That was demonstrated recently in an experiment in which a group of college students allowed to listen to music during final exams had a substantially lesser increase in blood pressure than a group *not* allowed the same musical advantage. The group accompanied by music also scored better (*Preventive Medicine*, March, 1979).

If classical music is not your style, go pop. There is no such thing as good or bad taste in something as intensely personal as music.

31/

Vacations: How about Making Your Next One an Adventure in Fitness?

How relaxing are vacations?

That depends on where you go, how you go, and why you go. If by going on a vacation you're looking to escape unfinished business, your chances of getting a good rest are not good.

"A vacation can be a wonderful celebration leading to rediscoveries of the body, forgotten skills, and social charms." Or it can be an unscheduled rendezvous with the very anxieties you had hoped to leave behind. That warning comes from Stephen A. Shapiro, Ph.D., and Alan J. Tuckman, M.D., authors of *Time Off: A Psychological Guide to Vacations* (Doubleday, 1978). It is very important to embark on a vacation in a proper frame of mind, they say. Because no island in the world is secluded enough to get you away from yourself.

So step number one in getting off on a good vacation is to make sure your home is reasonably together. Step number two is to alot yourself enough time.

Studies have shown that for a vacation to be optimally beneficial, it should run for at least a week. The first two or three days are needed for adjustment to the new environment, Drs. Shapiro and Tuckman say. It isn't until the third or fourth day that truly therapeutic fun can begin. And sometimes it takes a little bit of effort.

It takes stepping outside of your normal personality and experimenting with variations of your self-image. Which means *being* a jerk on the dance floor if you feel like it. You're in Tahiti, remember, so there's little chance of hearing about it on Monday at work.

Drs. Shapiro and Tuckman also suggest giving some serious thought to the pros and cons of traveling with family. Do you really want to take along that much of your home environment? Or would the chance to lose yourself *totally* leave you feeling more refreshed? Vacations are a time for being selfish.

And what better way to be selfish than to improve yourself? A change in environment can be a very effective aid in behavior modification, say Drs. Tuckman and Shapiro, whether it's for starting up a good habit or finishing off 151 a bad one—like smoking, or drinking, or snacking between meals. The beauty of a vacation is that it can get you away from the pressures and situations that may be encouraging you to misbehave in the first place.

HDL Levels Climb Along with Mountaineers

High-density lipoproteins—HDLs—are components that scientists feel reduce chances of heart disease. Thirteen male mountaineers nearly doubled theirs just three weeks into an eight-week climb.

Scientists from the Baker Medical Research Institute in Melbourne, Australia, measured HDL levels in mountaineers before, during, and after a strenuous ascent of Mount Dunagiri in the Himalayas. And in just 21 days, HDL levels had risen an average of 92 percent in all of them.

The researchers think it was the exercise. But they also credit the "conditions," not the least of which was the excitement, which the scientists termed "mental stress."

The study, in the researchers' words, proved two things: first, that "HDL concentrations rise rapidly with strenuous exercise." And second, that "extraordinarily high HDL concentrations" *can* be achieved (*Atherosclerosis*, October, 1979).

We interpret this to mean that adventuring can be good for the heart, because it involves exercise and a kind of resolvable "stress" that (in the sporting world) goes by the name *challenge*.

Keep that in mind as you recreate this year, not just on your vacation, but all year round.

And what if you haven't got any bad habits?

Then go find some more good ones. A vacation can be an opportunity to break new ground—to try dogsledding the Alaskan wilds, or canoeing the Amazon. (Don't laugh. These vacations are available, and for less money than you may think. It's the two-week booze baths at the shore that can get expensive.)

There is a need in all of us, say Drs. Shapiro and Tuckman, to prove to ourselves that we could—if we had to—be just as rugged as our founding fathers. The need comes, they theorize, from a distant fear that we may have to "rough it" for real someday. Be that as it may, proving to yourself that you can raft the raging Colorado isn't a bad way of putting a little wind in your sails for life back at the office.

Take a look at the following "off the beaten path" possibilities. They come to us from the American Adventurer's Association.

Vacations That Let Your Body Expand Your Mind

United States

Hawaii. *All Around Hawaii:* Summer trips lasting 24 days are offered to persons 12 and older. Exploring Hawaii's oceans and mountains, participants learn to function completely alone or with the group. Several features of the island of Hawaii are explored, from the 13,000-foot summit of Mauna Loa to the tropical rain forests and the powerful Pacific. While backpacking on lava or navigating an outrigger canoe, participants learn by doing. Following a few days of physical conditioning, expert instruction is provided on topics such as first aid, search and rescue techniques, route-finding, and environmental awareness. Food and equipment are furnished. **Cost:** $896. **When:** May to August. **Contact:** Hawaii Bound, 825 Keeaumoku Street, Room 220, Kailua, HI 96814, U.S.A. Phone (808) 946-6502.

Alaska. *Dogsledding the Iditarod Trail:* Traveling as the Eskimos have for centuries, participants set off from Anchorage on dogsledding treks in the Alaskan wilderness. On trips of varying lengths group members learn from experienced mountaineers the arts of subsistence living and arctic survival. The route along the Iditarod Trail is illuminated by the aurora borealis. Trips are planned with the resources and skills of participants in mind. **Cost:** On request. **When:** January to March. **Contact:** Otis B. Driftwood, Adventures Unlimited, 8701 Kathleen, Anchorage, AK 99502, U.S.A.

Minnesota. *Winter Weekend Trip:* A weekend trip in the Nemadji State Forest offers cross-country skiing, dogsledding, and winter camping. The three-day trip explores a wild and isolated section of the state about 150 miles north of the Twin Cities, a region of mixed hardwoods and pines. Many trails and old logging roads provide excellent dogsledding and cross-country skiing. A cabin is used for base camp, and heated arctic trail tents are provided for camping. Winter wildlife is plentiful in the beautiful and undisturbed environment. The group is limited to ten people who should have basic cross-country skiing experience. **Cost:** $90. **When:** February. **Contact:** Lynx Track Winter Travel, 5375 Eureka Road, Excelsior, MN 55331, U.S.A. Phone (612) 474-5190.

Montana. *Canoeing Historic Waters:* The Missouri River, once frequented by keelboats and steamboats when it was the principal pioneer route to the Northwest, is the waterway for guided and self-guided canoe trips of varying lengths. Canoeists put in at Fort Benton, Montana, the beginning of the Mullan Trail, and can paddle as far as Kipp State Park, a 160-mile stretch of river which was once a major gold rush route. Along the banks, monuments and landmarks document the river's rich history. Pickup service from Kipp State Park or upriver is available. **Cost:** $54 to $75 depending on trip length includes canoe, gear, pickup. **When:** May to September. **Contact:** Missouri River Cruises, Inc., Box 1212, Fort Benton, MT 59442, U.S.A. Phone (406) 622-3295.

Florida. *Key Scuba Adventures:* From a resort at Windley Key, divers enjoy waters with temperatures of 70°F in winter and visibility of 60 to 110 feet. Stretching 220 miles, the reef has depths ranging from 12 to 80 feet and is home to more than 600 species of tropical fish and 50 varieties of coral. Groups of four to ten can take four-day diving trips that include accommodations, three half-day dives, tank, weightbelts, and air. In addition to various package trips, guided dives with licensed captains, drive-it-yourself dive boats, and complete equipment rental and sales are available. Divers may investigate the area's many sunken Spanish galleons and World War II wrecks; more than half of all the gold lost in maritime disasters is estimated to be lying on the ocean floor off of the coast of Florida. Though services are geared toward certified divers, lessons in a freshwater pool are also offered. **Cost:** $16 to $25 a day depending on size of group, duration of stay, type of equipment provided; meals extra. **When:** Year-round excluding holidays. **Contact:** Coral Reef Resort, Box 575, Islamorada, FL 33036, U.S.A. Phone (305) 664-4955.

Abroad

Nepal. *Annapurna Trek:* Travelers ride elephants, visit with villagers, and trek at altitudes up to ten thousand feet during a 23-day expedition to study the cultural and natural features of Nepal. The trip begins with a flight from the United States to Kathmandu via Delhi. Highlights include an 11-day trek to explore the Annapurna region of central Nepal, with porters carrying the gear, a three-day raft trip on the Trisuli River, and a three-day visit to Royal Chitawan National Park to view wildlife. Trekkers have opportunities to visit religious shrines, cultural centers, and bazaars in the Kathmandu Valley, as well as to study geology and plants in a Himalayan setting. Accommodations are mostly in tent camps, with a few nights spent in lodges and hotels. The trip ends with a return flight from Delhi. **Cost:** $1,490 from Kathmandu includes land transportation, accommodations, meals (except in Kathmandu), guide. **When:** March, October. **Contact:** Nature Expeditions International, 599 College Avenue, Palo Alto, CA 94306, U.S.A. Phone (415) 328-6572.

This list merely scratches the surface of what's available. For more you can write to the American Adventurer's Association, Suite 301, 444 NE Ravenna Boulevard, Seattle, WA 98115. They've compiled a catalog entitled the *1981 Worldwide Adventure Travel Guide* (American Adventurer's Association, 1981).

32/

How to Relax in a Pinch

About 70 years ago, a young graduate student from Harvard had a profound insight. When we're under mental stress, we tense our muscles; and by tensing our muscles, we cause ourselves physical discomfort that tends to make our mental stress even worse. His name was Edmund Jacobson, M.D., and he went on to become a renowned physician who gradually perfected a technique for breaking this tense-mind, tense-muscle cycle. He called it progressive relaxation.

The technique has been enjoying something of a resurgence lately in these troubled times of ours. Psychologists and psychiatrists have been having luck treating such stress-related disorders as headaches, ulcers, high blood pressure, and colitis with the technique (or adaptations of it).

How does it work? By forcing us to focus in on how it actually *feels* to be physically relaxed.

Daily sessions lasting about 20 minutes are normally recommended, but once people get good at it, the sessions can be shortened and used in certain spur-of-the-moment situations—in a traffic jam or to cure pre-big-meeting jitters, for example.

If you're interested in learning the technique from an instructor, check with a psychologist or psychiatrist who is qualified to teach it. But you can also learn it from us. Sharon Faelten, a friend of mine, was taught a version of the technique, found it valuable, and gives the following account of how to go about it.

Take a comfortable position either sitting in a chair with your hands resting in your lap, or lying down on your back with your feet against a wall or heavy piece of furniture. Close your eyes.

Make a tight fist with your right hand, tensing the muscles in your wrist and forearm as you do. Hold tight for about five seconds, feeling the tension. Then unclench your fist, letting the tension drain from your forearm, wrist, and fingers. Note the difference between how your arm feels now and how it felt when it was tense. Repeat.

Now allow your right forearm and hand to remain relaxed while you clench your left fist and tense your left forearm. Note the difference between how your left arm feels and your relaxed arm feels. Now let your left arm relax, feeling the tension slowly drain out through your fingertips.

Next, tense your upper arms and shoulders. Hold a few seconds, then relax, again noting the difference between how your muscles feel when tense and how they feel when relaxed.

Now tense your neck. (It's probably the tensest part of your body.) Hold for a few seconds, then relax. At this point, your entire upper body should feel considerably more at ease than before you started.

Now make a frown, scowling as hard as you can. Relax. Try to feel the tension drain out of your eyes, cheeks, and lips.

Rise up on your toes (or push against the wall if lying down) to create some tension in your legs. Hold for a few seconds, then relax. Again, try to notice the tension drain away. Now your entire body should feel more at peace.

Your breathing all the while should be normal and rhythmic. Upon conclusion, though, take a deep breath, feeling the tension in your chest. Exhale. Breathe in again, hold, and let out, saying to yourself as you do, "I'm calm." Repeat once or twice. Concentrate on how calm you are. Relish the sense of well-being throughout your entire body.

Now picture yourself in the woods on a pleasant day. The light is just breaking through the trees, and as you take in the sights and sounds around you, you feel at peace with the world. (At this point, you may use whatever image conjures up feelings of tranquillity for you—perhaps a beach at sunset or a meadow filled with wild flowers.)

To conclude the exercise, slowly count to four. At one, you will begin to discard some of the deeper feelings of relaxation. At two, you are slightly more alert. At three, you will soon be ready to think and be fully alert. And at four, you may open your eyes.

If it sounds like self-hypnosis, it's not. Because levels of concentration are not as deep. And the mental focus with this procedure is on just that: relaxation. With hypnosis, the focus can be on anything from improving your tennis game to giving up gin and tonics.

The theory behind progressive relaxation is a good one—namely, that how we feel physically has much to do with how we think, emote, and act. When we come home at night with a headache, for example, how easy it is to find fault with what's for dinner. Progressive relaxation tries to teach us to recognize what tranquillity feels like on a muscular level—with the hope that that feeling will have a positive influence on what's going on inside our minds. If you'd like to learn more about Dr. Jacobson's theories, consult the following books:

Jacobson, Edmund. *Anxiety and Tension Control.* Philadelphia: J. B. Lippincott, 1964.

———. *Modern Treatment of Tense Patients.* Springfield, Ill.: Charles C. Thomas, 1970.

———. *You Must Relax.* New York: McGraw-Hill, 1976.

PART III/
HOW FITNESS FIGHTS DISEASE

The Ultimate Healer Is You

It isn't much fun to think about getting sick. Which is probably why not many of us do it. We probably learned very early, in fact, not to worry too much about our health. Because hypochondria, fifty thousand years ago, was apt to have put limitations on the aggressiveness it took to survive.

But in the following chapters we'll be talking a *lot* about health problems, both major diseases and minor conditions. Yet it's going to be a very positive discussion, because with all of these illnesses we're going to be emphasizing the element of *prevention*. Medical science has done its job of curing the infectious diseases that used to be our major killers. The diseases that remain are the ones that are now up to *us* to cure by not getting them in the first place. Heart disease, diabetes, strokes, and, to a degree, even cancer are all very much related to what the medical profession calls "lifestyle factors": obesity, smoking, inactivity, faulty eating habits, and stress.

Several years ago I attended a "wellness" conference in Clearwater, Florida. Keynote speaker William Hettler, M.D., of the University of Wisconsin, explained in his opening address that if suddenly a pill were developed that could cure all types of cancer, it would extend the average life expectancy in this country by about two years. If, on the other hand, each one of us would follow seven basic health practices, the average life expectancy could be increased by *11½ years*.

That's the kind of control we have. The seven practices Dr. Hettler mentioned were nothing out of reach: abstaining from tobacco, being within 20 percent of normal weight, getting some form of regular physical exercise, eating breakfast, avoiding unhealthful between-meal snacks, drinking in moderation, and getting about eight hours of sleep a night.

But whether or not these practices should be followed to the letter was not Dr. Hettler's point. His point was that a reasonably healthful lifestyle may be as close as we're going to get to the miracle cure we've all been waiting for —because by keeping ourselves healthy, we keep disease at bay.

Bear that in mind as you read through the following chapters. We should consider it very good news, indeed, that if there's an ultimate healer, that healer is in us.

33

Heart Disease: It Doesn't Deserve to Be Number One

We should consider ourselves lucky: Heart disease is still our number one killer, but 9 of its 11 major risk factors are within our power to control. The only ones we *can't* do anything about are family history and age. And those might not be as important as previously thought, anyway.

"I am not convinced that heredity, as a primary risk factor, is important. Nobody has yet come up with convincing evidence to show that your parents' history of heart disease or stroke has a direct bearing on your own."

Those encouraging words come from Risteard Mulcahy, M.D., former president of the Irish Heart Foundation and current head of the Heart Disease Research Unit at Saint Vincent's Hospital in Dublin. In his book, *Beat Heart Disease* (Arco, 1979), he notes also that atherosclerosis (the cause of over 80 percent of adult heart disease in Western countries) is "not part of the natural aging process and there is no reason why a healthy man of 80 should not have clear and atheroma-free arteries."

So why do more than half of us in this country succumb to some form of heart disease?

Because too many of us remain either ignorant of or indifferent to its cause. Heart disease is a much more controllable problem than its ranking as our number one killer would suggest. That it stops as many of us as it does, in fact, might be viewed as a source of embarrassment as much as remorse.

Varying combinations of the following *controllable* factors may place you in a high-risk category:

- cigarette smoking,
- obesity,
- high blood pressure,
- high ratio of LDL to HDL in serum cholesterol,
- high triglyceride levels,
- inactivity,
- diabetes,
- diet high in sugar and fat,
- stress.

We say varying combinations because it is unusual for any of these risk factors to be present on its own. Each has a way of either directly or indirectly giving rise to another. Which, depending on how you look at it, can be good news or bad.

We prefer to look at it as good news. Because what it means is that heart disease is like a house of cards: Eliminate one risk factor, and others fall. Say, for example, you decide to pull out inactivity . . .

By being more active, you're apt to lose weight, which may lower your blood pressure, *and* improve your serum cholesterol profile, *and* lower your blood sugar levels and blood fats—all of which is apt to make you feel better, and perhaps less stressed. And that may even reduce your desire to smoke.

Or let's say you decide to clean up your diet. That, too, is apt to result in weight loss—and, hence, lower blood pressure, a better cholesterol profile, reduced blood sugar, lower triglycerides, and perhaps an improved ability to handle stress.

The point is, the risk factors for heart disease are one big not-so-happy family. And, by insulting one, you stand to slight the rest.

The reverse, however, is also true. Admit one, and you risk entertaining the entire clan. Stress, for example, can encourage cigarette smoking, which can raise blood pressure, which can exacerbate high cholesterol levels, which can be made worse by a fatty diet, which can elevate triglycerides, which can again raise blood pressure, which can make you feel stressed, which can increase your desire to smoke—and around you go again. Only this time with even graver results.

Scientists call that kind of cycle a closed-feedback loop. And it can be literally murder.

"An understanding of the causes of heart disease and the intelligent application of preventive measures could, I believe, lead to virtual elimination of heart disease and stroke . . . for people under 65 or 70 years old." Dr. Mulcahy is adamant about that, and indeed there are statistics to back him up. The frequency of coronary heart disease in the United States has fallen by about 20 percent over the past eight years—a reflection, he assures us, of the efficacy of our recent bent toward fitness.

So which of heart disease's risk factors should you decide to attack?

Only you can say, because only you know which you are guilty of. And only you know which is going to be easiest for you to defeat. We hope the accompanying table will help you. It's a family tree of sorts, showing where the ties between risk factors lie.

Good luck. And keep in mind that whichever risk factor you choose to attack, there are others that are going to be feeling your wrath.

Heart Disease Risk Factors: Causes and Treatments

Risk Factor	May Give Rise to or Worsen the Effects of	May Be Relieved by
Cigarette smoking	High blood pressure High LDL-to-HDL ratios High triglyceride levels Inactivity Stress	Cessation of smoking
Obesity (being more than 20 percent over ideal weight)	High blood pressure High LDL-to-HDL ratios High triglyceride levels Inactivity High blood sugar Stress	Exercise, improvement of diet (less fat, more unrefined carbohydrates)
High blood pressure	Stress High LDL-to-HDL ratios High triglyceride levels High blood sugar	Exercise, weight loss, cessation of smoking, alleviation of stress, improvement of diet (decrease salt)
High LDL-to-HDL ratios	High blood pressure High triglyceride levels High blood sugar	Exercise, weight loss, cessation of smoking, improvement of diet
High triglyceride levels	High blood pressure High LDL-to-HDL ratios High blood sugar	Exercise, weight loss, cessation of smoking, improvement of diet, alleviation of stress
Inactivity	Obesity High blood pressure High LDL-to-HDL ratios High triglyceride levels High blood sugar Stress	Exercise
High blood sugar	High triglyceride levels	Exercise, weight loss
Faulty diet	Obesity High blood pressure High LDL-to-HDL ratios High triglyceride levels Inactivity High blood sugar Stress	Improvement of diet
Stress	Cigarette smoking Obesity High blood pressure High LDL-to-HDL ratios High triglyceride levels High blood sugar, faulty diet	Exercise, cessation of smoking

NOTE: HDL, or high-density lipoproteins, is that fraction of cholesterol considered protective against heart disease. LDL, or low-density lipoproteins, is that cholesterol fraction considered harmful. A high proportion of HDL to LDL is desirable.

34/

Cancer: What You *Can* Do

Will you die of cancer?

That's a question, fortunately, that no one can answer better than you can. Because despite the environmental odds that continue to stack up against us, research affirms that the upper hand against cancer is still ours.

"The major causal factors so far identified in human cancer relate to personal habits and lifestyle," says John Higginson, M.D., director of the International Agency for Research on Cancer.

This is not to say that air pollution and pesticides do not play their roles. They do. But compared to smoking cigarettes, and eating a disordered diet, and allowing yourself to be inactive or depressed, the risks posed by your polluted environment are actually quite small.

Take lung cancer, for example. Lung cancer in 1978 accounted for almost *one-fourth* of all cancer deaths in this country.

Air pollution, you say?

No. Cigarettes.

Smoking is responsible for an estimated 97 percent of all lung cancers in men and 74 percent in women, according to *American Scientist* (July/August, 1981). The smoker who campaigns against air pollution in light of these statistics would seem to be fuming in the wrong direction.

Many of us tend to pass the buck with other forms of cancer as well. Tumors of the digestive organs, for example, killed more people in 1978 than any other form of cancer. But not because of food additives.

Harry B. Demopoulos, M.D., of the New York University Medical Center puts the blame on "disordered nutrition": too much food, too much fat, too little fiber, and deficiencies in vitamin A.

"Diet is important," agrees Gio B. Gori, Ph.D., formerly of the National Cancer Institute. In view of its recognized role in cancer, diet has been linked to more than half of *all* cancers in women, and at least one-third of all cancers in men.

If these statistics sound grim, they are not. Because what they boil down to is this: Our two deadliest forms of cancer (those of the digestive and respiratory tracts) are due largely to factors (diet and smoking) which are very much within our power to control.

162

What about the occupational hazards of working around toxic chemicals, asbestos, and radiation?

They exist. But they, too, can be reduced by living a more healthful lifestyle. Asbestos workers who smoke, for example, increase their chances of getting lung cancer 90 times over the risk of men who neither smoke nor work with asbestos (*Journal of the American Medical Association*, August 3, 1979). And in an English study on the effects of air pollution from burning coal, it was found that while smokers were getting more lung cancer, nonsmokers were not.

Why should this be?

One theory is that smoking damages a mechanism the lungs have for clearing themselves of chemicals that may do damage to other parts of the body. Which may be why heavy smokers—in addition to increasing their chances of getting lung cancer *thirtyfold*—also get more cancers of the throat, mouth, pancreas, kidneys, and bladder than do nonsmokers.

Which is why it's so important to establish a well-rounded defence, an important part of which, says Claus Bahnson, Ph.D., is a healthy attitude. Dr. Bahnson warns that feelings of depression and despair can upset the body's production of hormones, and the immune system as a result. "People who are very rigid, and use denial and repression, and lack awareness of their emotions" also appear to be more prone to the disease, Dr. Bahnson says.

The mental factor is a considerable one. It can weaken the defenses of the depressed. But it can also strengthen the defenses of the vibrant. In this regard it may be your most important weapon of all, particularly if you know there's been a history of cancer in your family. If you have reason to think you *are* genetically susceptible, work it to your advantage—by being all that much more dedicated to the anticancer lifestyle we've outlined (see the following box). *Don't* let your susceptibility depress you.

Where does physical fitness figure into an anticancer lifestyle?

You can't run away from cancer as effectively as you can heart disease. But there *is* evidence that exercise is worth the effort. Dr. Gori advises it as a way of stabilizing weight—and hence the integrity of immune systems that obesity can undermine. "People should have a regular schedule of exercise commensurate with their age and physical capabilities," he says. (When applied to mice by researchers at the Labor Science Research Institute in Japan, this prescription did quite nicely. Mice restricted from exercise developed cancer at a rate of 60 percent, whereas mice made to exercise on a treadmill developed the disease at a rate of only 23.5 percent. The exercise group also ate less and proved more resistant to the carcinogen benzidine.)

So stop feeling helpless against cancer. "Since 1950 . . . despite long-standing industrialization, a rapidly expanding petrochemical industry, and increasing awareness of occupational hazards, the overall cancer rates are decreasing in both black and white females and in white males if tumors related

The Anticancer Lifestyle

Avoid the enemy:

- Cigarettes. Smoking a pack of cigarettes a day puts your chances of lung cancer at one out of ten (30 times greater than the nonsmoker's).
- Fatty foods. A high-fat diet is suspected of upsetting the body's hormone balance, thus contributing to breast cancer.
- Food additives. Red Dye number 40, sodium nitrite, and saccharin appear to be the worst offenders. Check labels and avoid them when possible.
- Contaminated water. If you have reason to believe your water is impure, have it tested for dangerous levels of: arsenic, cadmium, chromium, lead, nickel, asbestos, radioactivity.
- Heavy consumption of alcohol. Heavy drinking, especially of hard liquor, increases the risk of mouth, throat, larynx, esophageal, and liver cancers. Consider anything over the equivalent of 28 drinks a week to be heavy.
- X-rays. Always question the need for an x-ray. Breast self-examination is an acceptable alternative to much mammography screening, and many dental x-rays are unnecessary.
- Overexposure to sunlight. We'll define overexposure as more than about 20 minutes a day of direct sunlight, or a burn, whichever comes first. Too much sun increases risk of skin cancer.
- Air pollution. The risks appear marginal, but worth avoiding nonetheless. Try not to exercise around really heavy traffic. Or if presented with an option of relocating, take into consideration the amount of industry in a prospective area. Asbestos, smelting, and petrochemical plants deserve a particularly wide berth.
- Stress. A little bit can be good. But a lot can be bad. Why? Because there have been studies indicating a link between chronic

to alcohol and tobacco are excluded," reports Dr. Higginson in the *Journal of the National Cancer Institute* (December, 1979).

Cancer, in other words, is not the environmental monster we sometimes think it is. And the sooner we realize this, the better, because a "what's the use" attitude leads to a "what's the use" lifestyle. And that *can* be deadly

stress and cancer-causing hormonal imbalances. What's more, stress tends to encourage smoking, drinking, poor digestion, sleeping problems, and emotional disorders—all of which can weaken your natural defenses.

Bolster your defenses:

- Get all your vitamins. "Chronic deficiencies of vitamins A, vitamin E, and selenium have been shown to increase the susceptibility of animals to chemically induced tumors," reports Gio B. Gori, Ph.D. So if your diet is lacking, consider supplementation.
- Eat plenty of fiber. Fiber inhibits bowel cancer by speeding transit time and cutting in half the amount of time some potential carcinogens are in contact with the intestinal lining.
- Eat less. "Of all dietary modifications," Dr. Gori says, "caloric restriction has had the most regular influence on tumor formation. With few exceptions, caloric restriction generally has an inhibiting effect." Avoiding foods high in calories but low in nutrients (such as sugar, bleached flour, and fats) is your best way of cutting back.
- Go heavy on vegetables. Vegetables contain enzymes that appear to inhibit cancer growth. The most effective seem to be beans, broccoli, cabbage, and cauliflower.
- Exercise. It makes you stronger physically as well as emotionally. And it also keeps your weight down. Studies show that obese women are at a greater risk of developing breast cancer than women of normal weight.
- Keep your chin up. "If deaths from lung cancer are subtracted," one researcher has observed, "the overall incidence of death from cancer would be less today than in 1939—about 10 percent less." The cancer epidemic, in other words, may be overrated. So stop thinking of it as the "Big C."

35/

Diabetes: Stop Asking for It

Not to scare you, but if you're inactive, overweight, and over 40, your chances of having diabetes are considerable.

But wait a minute. Isn't diabetes that rare blood disease that people have to take insulin for?

Not in most cases. There are *two* types of diabetes: One requires taking insulin and affects only about 1 out of every 450 Americans; the other, however, may not require insulin and is far more common—about ten times more common, in fact. The American Diabetes Association estimates that some form of diabetes will affect one out of ten Americans at some point in their lives. And the older—and fatter—we get, the more susceptible we become. Forty to 60 percent of people over 80 have diabetes.

Diabetes: A Disease on the Rise

As this graph shows, the prevalence of diabetes rose over 600 percent in approximately one generation—from 1935 to 1978.

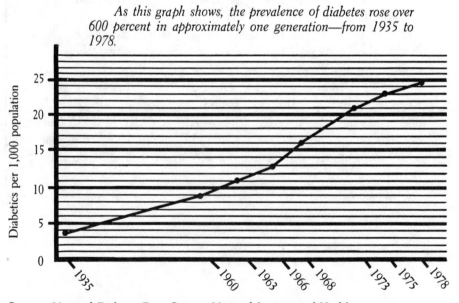

Source: National Diabetes Data Group—National Institutes of Health.

Currently, diabetes ranks as our number three killer, and it's a disease on the rise (see accompanying graph). The total number of diabetics in this country has doubled in the past 15 years, and incidence of the disease continues to escalate at an annual rate of 5 percent.

What's the problem?

The way we live, for one thing. In an estimated 80 percent of all cases of diabetes, obesity—and perhaps inactivity and bad diet—play major roles. To a large degree, diabetes is a disease brought on by lifestyle.

How does it work?

Diabetes affects the way our bodies use blood sugar, the basic fuel for all bodily functions.

In Type 1 diabetes (the rare kind, usually beginning during childhood or adolescence), the pancreas produces too little of the hormone insulin, which is responsible for putting blood sugar to work. As a result, the blood sugar (glucose) that should be fueling bodily functions wanders about troublesomely in the bloodstream. Treatment of Type 1 diabetes involves regular doses of insulin to put this blood sugar to proper use.

Type 2 (also called noninsulin-dependent and maturity-onset diabetes) is not so simple. People with this form of the disease produce insulin, sometimes even too much, but the insulin (for reasons not yet fully understood) doesn't do the job of putting blood sugar to work. And so, as with Type 1 diabetes, the result is a surplus of glucose in the blood, the dangers of which are numerous and potentially grave. Chronically high levels of sugar in the blood increase risks of atherosclerosis (hardening of the arteries), kidney disease, and stroke, and can directly cause blindness, nerve damage, and gangrene. Indeed, diabetes is a disease that, because it strikes at the body's ability to energize itself, can have far-reaching and very debilitating results.

So what can be done about diabetes?

Type 1, which usually manifests itself obviously and early in life, is most effectively treated by regular doses of insulin.

Type 2, however, is best treated by controlling the factors that seem to encourage its onset in the first place: inactivity, bad diet, and excess weight. Granted, there may be genetic and perhaps even viral factors at play in Type 2's prevalence, but Type 2 diabetes is rare in countries where people eat wisely and exercise. Studies show that a person's chances of developing Type 2 double with every 20 pounds he or she is overweight.

With that in mind, may we suggest the following two measures for diabetes prevention. And if we're beginning to sound like a broken record ("exercise and eat a good diet"), we're not sorry. We're glad, in fact (and you should be, too), that science is finding out that some of our most complex illnesses can be prevented by relatively simple means.

Exercise

From studies of how exercise affects the body's ability to use blood sugar, it appears that our metabolisms are as capable of getting "out of shape" as the rest of us. Muscle cells, through disuse, seem to lose their ability to respond to insulin. And it is insulin, remember, that puts blood sugar to work. Reporting on a study done at Yale University, Vijay R. Soman, M.D., writes in the *New England Journal of Medicine* (November 29, 1979) that "physical training can be valuable in the treatment of obesity and maturity-onset [Type 2] diabetes because it augments tissue sensitivity to insulin."

Dr. Soman studied the effects of physical training on six previously untrained, healthy men. The men were made to exercise for an hour at a time on stationary bicycles four times a week, and even though the men's body weights did not change, their sugar uptake by insulin was increased by 30 percent after six weeks of training. What exercise seems to do is increase the number of "receptor sites" on muscle cells (to which insulin can bind), thus facilitating the uptake of blood sugar as a result.

Diet

So exercise regulates blood sugar by keeping muscle cells in shape to use it. There's another approach to keeping blood sugar levels normal, though, and that's simply not to flood the blood with sugar in the first place. Some researchers feel that inordinate amounts of refined sugar in the American diet may in time actually desensitize the pancreas. And it's the job of the pancreas, remember, to produce enough insulin to keep blood sugar from rising to unhealthy levels. So step number one in putting your diet to work against diabetes is:

Eat fewer foods containing refined sugar. Far better sources of energy are complex carbohydrate foods, such as grains, beans, and potatoes. And to satisfy your sweet tooth, reach for fruit, which contains a form of sugar (fructose) that does not cause as rapid a rise in blood sugar as glucose. Step number two:

Eat less fat. Fat is bad for two reasons. First, its nine calories per gram (carbohydrates and protein contain only about four) can contribute to obesity, which is the single "most powerful risk factor for diabetes," according to the World Health Organization. Second, high blood fats increase the likelihood of plaque buildup in the tiny lesions (cracks) in arteries that studies are now beginning to suggest *too much blood sugar may cause.* So our sugar-laden, high-fat diets have diabetes and heart disease going hand in hand. Sugar pits our arteries, and fat encourages the filling of these pits with plaque. Step number three:

Eat more fiber. Fiber has the ability to slow the rate at which sugar enters the bloodstream, and it also has some ability to decrease the bloodstream's absorption of fat. Research shows that diabetics put on high-fiber diets (rich in whole grains, vegetables, and fruits) are able to reduce their insulin doses dramatically. Step number four:

Eat foods rich in chromium. Studies show that for insulin to be effective it must be in the company of adequate amounts of the trace mineral chromium. The mineral, however, is one dangerously lacking in the average high-fat, sugar-rich American diet. Recent investigations have led to the recommendation that we ingest between 50 and 200 micrograms of chromium a day—perhaps more if our diets are excessively high in sugar. Brewer's yeast is an excellent source of the mineral, as are whole wheat products (another reason to eat more fiber), mushrooms, chili peppers, and the other foods listed in the accompanying table.

Selected Sources of Chromium

	Chromium Content
Brewer's yeast Liver	Excellent
Potatoes, with skin Beef Vegetables, fresh Bread, whole grain Cheese Chicken legs	Good
Fruit, fresh Chicken breast Fish and seafood	Fair
Spaghetti, white Corn flakes Milk, skim Butter Margarine Sugar	Poor

SOURCE: Adapted from "Mineral Elements: New Perspectives," by Walter Mertz (*Journal of the American Dietetic Association*, September, 1980).

So there you have it: how not to get diabetes. If you've been exercising regularly and eating wisely already, keep up the good work. But if you haven't, you might want to consider diabetes one more reason to start.

36/

Depression: A Natural Reaction to Stress

The human spirit may be indomitable. But it's also human. It periodically needs time off to regain its strength. And the sooner millions of us realize that, the better. Ronald R. Fieve, M.D., a psychiatrist from New York City and author of *Moodswing: The Third Revolution in Psychiatry* (Bantam, 1976), estimates that between 15 and 20 percent of the adult population suffers from some form of depression.

Perhaps the rich more than the poor, though. And the ambitious more than the lazy. Indeed, Horatio Alger might not have been happy to know that psychiatrists would one day call depression an "illness of success."

Why should success be depressing?

For the same reason failure is: It's a source of stress. It forces us to look at who we are, where we are going, *why* we are going—and whether or not we *deserve* to be going. If it makes you feel any better, Abraham Lincoln, Theodore Roosevelt, and Winston Churchill all had recurrent bouts with depression.

They rose above it, however, as we all can. Depression, in fact, can—and should—be viewed as a kind of pit-stop, "an opportunity for a person not just to learn more about himself, but to become more whole than he was," says Frederic F. Flach, M.D., in *The Secret Strength of Depression* (J. B. Lippincott, 1974).

"It is time that we recognize the ubiquity and contagiousness of depression," Dr. Flach points out, "and realize that depression is not only a highly common way of reacting to stress—a reaction that sometimes requires medical attention—but that, when acknowledged, it is also for millions a unique opportunity to redefine themselves and resolve long-standing destructive conflicts within themselves and their environment." Depression, in other words, can provide us—as its name implies—with an impetus to spring back. *If* we learn how to handle it.

Chronic vs. Acute Depression

Depression comes in two forms: acute and chronic. Acute depression can
170 be the result of a run-in with your boss, a fight with your spouse, a smack-up

with your car, the death of someone close to you. An acute depression, in other words, is one that has a specific and identifiable cause and is appropriate to the severity of that cause.

Chronic depression, on the other hand, may seem inappropriate to the severity of its cause—because it may appear not to have one. It is the result of acute depressions that have been allowed to build up to the point of obscuring themselves. Its symptoms may include insomnia, fatigue, low self-esteem, withdrawal, difficulty in making decisions, and a tendency to put things off. And it may be difficult to identify, Dr. Flach points out, because it may seem part of a person's temperament rather than a passing mood.

Perhaps the most important difference between acute and chronic depression, though, is that whereas acute depressions are usually unavoidable, chronic depression is to be avoided at all costs.

"In contrast to acute depression, which affords an opportunity for insight, chronic depression is nearly always disabling and will complicate a person's life in ways that may be hard to correct and may at times be irreversible," Dr. Flach warns. Which is why we must deal with our acute depressions *as they come*, and not allow them to become chronic.

How?

Psychologically, by forcing ourselves to confront and analyze our acute depressions, as painful as that might be.

Even Fun Can Get Us Down

Why?

Because fun is a source of stress. Another attack on the central nervous system. Another weight to slightly alter our delicate psychological equilibrium. Depression is a form of psychobiological (mental and physical) fatigue. And anything grandly out of the ordinary runs a risk of producing it.

"If, for example," says Frederic F. Flach, M.D., "a man receives an important promotion, is transferred to a new part of the country, . . . and attends the college graduation of his only child, all in a few months' time, he is likely to become somewhat depressed."

Psychobiologically pooped, in other words.

"His reaction may well be puzzling to himself and others because most of these changes could generally be thought of as good." But "a series of changes, for better or worse, compacted into a small enough span of time, is apt to produce depression in most people."

Keep that in mind the next time you feel a little guilty for feeling blue following a fantastic weekend or a power-packed vacation with the family. Your body (and mind) may simply be recoiling from the shock.

To do that, most psychiatrists and psychologists suggest making it a point to talk to somebody—be it a spouse, a friend, or a professional counselor—at the very onset of a depressed feeling. Even if it makes the experience more painful, depression is best confronted *directly* and *early*. And the insight that an outside opinion can afford is often exactly what is needed to put an acute depression in proper perspective. We must learn to keep in touch with our emotions "on a day-to-day basis," says Dr. Flach. And we must learn to be flexible and imaginative to keep from being unduly hurt by setbacks that are, after all, the price we pay for being ambitious.

What we can do physically to avoid chronic depression may be even more encouraging. Studies are showing that for many people, chronic depression appears to be caused by a change in brain chemistry. A change that is treatable by nutrition.

The Difference Nutrition Can Make

"Studies of the neurophysiological operations of the brain point up the tendency of the depressed person to show alterations in the metabolism of substances . . . that affect the transmission of impulses within the nervous system," says Dr. Flach. One of these substances is serotonin. And what's being found to aid in its production is tryptophan (an amino acid in protein) and vitamins B_6 and niacin.

Harvey Ross, M.D., author of *Hypoglycemia: The Disease Your Doctor Won't Treat* (Pinnacle, 1980), routinely recommends a good B complex vitamin—two or three times a day after meals—for most of his patients suffering from depression. "To be any more specific about dosages is difficult," he said, "because everybody is different."

Two more nutrients thought to play a role in depressioon are calcium and magnesium. August F. Daro, M.D., an obstetrician and gynecologist from Chicago, recently told us of the success he's been having in treating his depressed patients (premenstrual women, especially) with 200 milligrams of magnesium and 400 milligrams of calcium daily.

Diet may also help resolve depression, particularly in light of the fact that "depressed people generally don't eat well," as one M.D. has pointed out. It's thought that loss of appetite, and the nutritional deficiencies that accompany it, may be a cause of depression as well as a symptom. Add to the depressed person's loss of appetite his tendency to abuse coffee and alcohol—both of which deplete the body of B vitamins—and the nutritional aspects of depression begin to look real, indeed.

What Exercise Can Do

Exercise may not be the answer to depression, but it's certainly a good way to put yourself in the right frame of mind to look for an answer. Scientists are discovering that vigorous exercise encourages the release of mood-elevating chemicals in the brain called *endorphins,* which are similar to morphine in their chemical makeup. They also resemble it in their effects, as anyone who's ever experienced a runner's high can gladly attest.

Depression may have the reputation for being a mental problem, but it needs all the physical help it can get. As the ancient Greeks discovered centuries ago, mind and body are in this thing together.

37/

Arthritis: Beat It
with Your Muscles
and Your Mind

If you don't have arthritis, you know someone who does. The disease afflicts one out of eight Americans.

"It comes to almost all of us who live long enough," says George E. Ehrlich, M.D., director of the Division of Rheumatology at the Hahnemann Medical College and Hospital in Philadelphia. "To a degree, it's a natural consequence of activities and time."

To a degree. There are people in their forties so crippled by the disease they can't work. And arthritic children who can't play. Arthritis is *not* just a disease of the aged.

It is a disease of the joints. It can take the form of minor stiffness—or excruciating pain. It can nag a single joint, or torture the entire body. Doctors have cataloged the disease into more than 100 forms. Osteoarthritis and rheumatoid arthritis are the most common.

Osteoarthritis is the gradual wearing away of the padding (cartilage) between weight-bearing bones. It can result from injury, misuse, or no use at all. Rheumatoid arthritis is less specific. It can attack connective tissue anywhere in the body—for what reason, however, no one knows.

Can arthritis be prevented? Maybe. Relieved? Yes. And doctors are finding that one of the best ways to keep joints healthy is to exercise them.

Joints need to move in order to breathe—not air, but "synovial" fluid, whose job it is to supply nourishment to the cartilage (living tissue) responsible for keeping bones working together smoothly. One rheumatologist has described this "feeding" process as a series of "intermittent compressions and releases by which synovial fluid enters and leaves the cartilage in very much the same way as air enters and leaves the lungs." And so what happens when we lay idle for too long is that cartilage begins to run dry.

But exercise does more than just feed cartilage; it guards it.

"By strengthening the muscles around a joint, you allow the joint to work as it was designed," Dr. Ehrlich explained. "Joints need muscles for support."

(That's why it's so important to warm up before exercising, Dr. Ehrlich says, particularly as we get older. A cold muscle is like a weak muscle; it permits bones to interact in ways that are unnaturally abrasive to the cartilage between them.)

Are some exercises better for warding off arthritis than others? we asked Dr. Ehrlich.

The kind of exercise you do, he said, makes less difference than how you do it. Whether you run, swim, play golf, play tennis, or ride a bike, the important thing is to do it right. Improper exercise can be worse than none at all.

Jogging? Some experts warn against it because of the stress it puts on hips and knees, but John Skosey, M.D., chief of the rheumatology section of the University of Illinois Hospital in Chicago, says that with the proper precautions, running is harmless. A good, smooth surface (preferably one that "gives"), good shoes, and some good stretching and warm-up exercises, he says, are the keys to pain-free running. (A study made of Finnish long-distance runners would seem to prove Dr. Skosey right: It showed that the runners had less osteoarthritis than a group of sedentaries used as a control.)

One of the biggest problems with arthritis, experts seem to agree, is that people tend to interpret its pains as a sign *not* to exercise. And so muscles around painful joints deteriorate, making matters even worse.

Too often, says Wanda Sadoughi, Ph.D., it's the same with sex. People with arthritic pain have sex less when they *ought* to have it more.

Dr. Sadoughi is the director of the Sex Dysfunction Clinic at Cook County Hospital in Chicago, and according to her, sex is one of the best analgesics going. "It could be any number of things," she said, "something biochemical or hormonal. The emotional aspect is obviously important. Sex is a wonderful source of self-esteem, a great reliever of stress, and pretty fair exercise, to boot."

The people who are having the most success against arthritis, it seems, are those using strategies a lot more pleasant than drugs.

Why?

Because there is a strong psychological element to arthritis, says John Baum, M.D., of the University of Rochester Medical School. Attitude can either reverse or accelerate the disease. People who take an active role in combating arthritis feel better mentally as well as physically. The most dangerous situation of all, Dr. Baum says, is when arthritis begins to cripple the spirit. It is perhaps the most insidious feature of the disease that it both creates and feeds on mental stress.

"We're finding that the most important thing of all in treating arthritis," Dr. Baum said, "is a patient's willingness to fight. People with serious deformities who refuse to give up do as well as patients with minimal illness but less desire."

That's nice to hear coming from a doctor, particularly since some of the drugs now being prescribed for arthritis are causing side effects as dangerous as the disease itself.

If you're being bothered by pain and stiffness you suspect may be arthritis, take action. Arthritis is a nasty disease, but it's also a coward. You stand to gain only by challenging it to something physical

38/

Bad Backs: Why Everybody's Got One

If it seems like just about everybody you talk to has a bad back, it's because just about everybody does. "Anyone who lives an average life span without suffering from backache belongs to a privileged minority," contends back expert Hamilton Hall, M.D., author of *The Back Doctor* (McGraw-Hill, 1980). Indeed, an estimated two-thirds of all adults suffer from back pain at some point during their lives.

Why are our backs so weak?

Because we were a little hasty in getting up off all fours. About four million years ago, someone's brain said, "I think I could get more done if I didn't have to use my hands as feet." And so up that person stood. And the rest of us followed. And our backs have been trying to catch up ever since.

Not that our backs are so archaic that we should be ashamed of them. The human spine is a wonderfully intricate structure. It's just that we are now asking it to function vertically when its basic design is still more suited for life on the horizontal. Indeed, virtually all common back problems are a result of downward pressure causing wear and tear on the bones of the spine (vertebrae) and the pads (disks) that separate them. Backache is a discouragingly "normal" development, Dr. Hall says.

So what do we do with these backs of ours that can lock up on us at the drop of a hat?

We learn to live with them, Dr. Hall says. We learn to sit, stand, bend, lift, sleep, brush our teeth, bowl, have sex, work, and give piggyback rides with them. Because in time, most back problems will cure themselves. Studies show, in fact, that backache is more of a *middle-age* than old-age problem. By the time we turn 60 or so, our backs usually have made do with the imperfections that can cripple us in our thirties.

With that in mind, surgery, Dr. Hall says, should be avoided at all costs. "Fewer than 5 percent of all people with back pain are likely to benefit from surgery," he reports. "At least 19 out of 20, including serious cases, are better off with some combination of physiotherapy, medication, exercise, and what we refer to as proper ADL—activities of daily living."

We'll explain those activities in a minute. But first we've got to determine what kind of back problem you have. Dr. Hall says all common backaches are due to one of the following:

- a worn facet joint (which he calls Type 1);
- a protruding disk (Type 2);
- a pinched nerve (Type 3);
- or, unfortunately, a combination of two of these, or even all three.

How can you tell which is you?

Type 1 back pain hurts most "when you arch your back, as you would when you lean back to look up at the ceiling," Dr. Hall says. The pain you feel is mainly at the top of your buttocks, and you find that bending slightly forwards tends to relieve it. "Your trouble begins with a minor incident of routine exertion, such as picking up a garden hoe or retrieving a golf ball," and it usually subsides, if you rest it, within 4 to 14 days. If you're Type 1, you probably experience such attacks two or three times a year.

Type 2 shares many of the symptoms of Type 1, but it also has these distinguishing differences, Dr. Hall says: "A Type 2 attack may begin with the same sort of incident as Type 1, but the onset of pain is likely to be less sharp and immediate; more often it will build up slowly, over a couple of days, from mild discomfort to severe pain. The pain will recede noticeably in a week or two but, unlike Type 1 pain, it won't disappear. Instead, it will linger on as a nagging backache or, in some cases, as an intense and constant pain." Unlike Type 1, though, Type 2 isn't aggravated more when you bend back; it's bending forward that intensifies the pain. "Like Type 1, Type 2 pain is felt mainly in the back, although it may radiate into the buttocks and legs," Dr. Hall explains, "just as Type 1 does."

Type 3 pain might be thought of as Type 2 Plus, Dr. Hall says, because it involves a disk that has protruded to the point of pressing on a nerve. Hence, it has many of the symptoms of Type 2 pain, but also some of its own: Pain can extend not just into the thighs, but lower—sometimes even to the feet and toes. Type 3 pain usually comes on over a day or two, builds, and stays for weeks. It is made distinctly worse by bending forward, and it is potentially the most serious of the three types because prolonged pressure can damage nerve function. It is also the least common, however, and is responsible for only about 10 percent of all back woes.

What causes these three types of back pain?

In the case of Type 1 pain, it's usually a disk (see figure 1) that has flattened to the point of allowing the bones of a facet joint to rub against one another. Disks can flatten because of a gradual drying-out process (a natural consequence of aging), and that process can be hastened by a life of hard

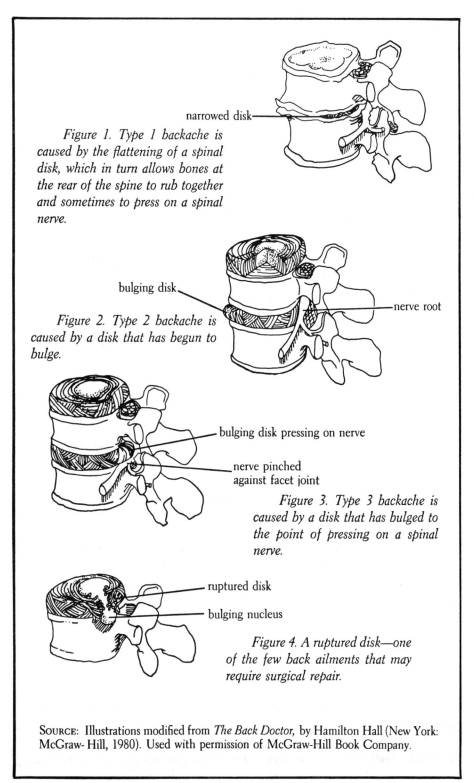

narrowed disk—

Figure 1. Type 1 backache is caused by the flattening of a spinal disk, which in turn allows bones at the rear of the spine to rub together and sometimes to press on a spinal nerve.

bulging disk

—nerve root

Figure 2. Type 2 backache is caused by a disk that has begun to bulge.

bulging disk pressing on nerve

nerve pinched against facet joint

Figure 3. Type 3 backache is caused by a disk that has bulged to the point of pressing on a spinal nerve.

ruptured disk

bulging nucleus

Figure 4. A ruptured disk—one of the few back ailments that may require surgical repair.

SOURCE: Illustrations modified from *The Back Doctor*, by Hamilton Hall (New York: McGraw-Hill, 1980). Used with permission of McGraw-Hill Book Company.

physical labor and heavy lifting. It can also be aggravated by bad posture, pregnancy, or a potbelly, because anything that causes you to arch your back causes facet joints (located at the rear of the spine) to press together.

Type 2 back pain is the result of a disk doing more bulging than collapsing, because disks are not "dead" tissue. They contain nerve fibers, and they hurt when they get pushed out of shape (see figure 2).

Type 3 back pain is the result of a disk bulging to the point of pressing on a spinal nerve (see figure 3). And if things really get tight, a disk can rupture (see figure 4)—one of the few cases in which surgery may be required for repair.

Maybe now you can see why bed rest is so often recommended as the first order of business following a back attack. By lying down, you relieve pressure on disks, which in turn relieves pressure on spinal nerves, which should, in turn, erase the reason for the muscles of your back going into painful—but *protective* —spasm. Muscle spasms are your body's way of encouraging the very immobilization you need in order to heal. And not until those spasms relax is it time to think about doing some corrective exercises—exercises, as strange as it may sound, that concentrate not on the back, but rather the stomach.

Why the stomach?

Because strong stomach muscles can provide a weak back with the additional support it needs. When stomach muscles are weak, greater pressure gets passed on to the disks, which are so important to spare.

Abdominal exercises, however, are not the entire answer to getting along with a bad back. As we mentioned earlier, there are those all-important ADLs —activities of daily living—as Dr. Hall calls them. The idea is to make life as easy on your back as possible *in as many situations as possible.*

How to Sleep

If you sleep on your back, roll a couple of pillows into a bolster to raise up your knees. Or if you prefer sleeping on your stomach, "try sleeping with a pillow under the front of your pelvis to reduce the sag in your lower back," Dr. Hall says. Side-sleepers should curl into a ball and place a pillow *between* their knees. The purpose of all of these positions is to reduce pressure on spinal disks.

How to Sit

Not for very long is the first rule of thumb. Because sitting can create a greater load on spinal disks than standing (see graph). You can reduce that load by making sure to support yourself with your elbows if you must lean forward to work at your desk. In other more recreational sitting situations, try to keep your feet raised—on either a step stool or a stack of books, and place a small pillow between the back of your chair and the area just above your buttocks.

How to Stand

"Never stand flat-footed if you can put one foot up on a stool or a low shelf —the posture drinkers assume at a stand-up bar. Saloon keepers discovered the comfort of this position long before doctors developed the theory behind it," Dr. Hall says.

How to Lift

With the back as straight as possible. Squat, in other words, but don't bend over. The more work you can pass on to the legs, the better. "The most hazardous lifts are the ones for which you are unprepared," warns Dr. Hall. And the most difficult, even when you *are* prepared, are the ones where you must hoist something over a barrier at arm's length, e.g., a 40-pound nephew out of a high-sided crib. Make it a habit to *think* before you attempt a lift. If even the thought of it hurts, chances are *it* will.

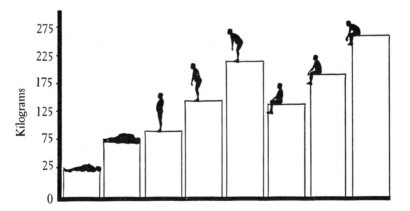

This graph illustrates the relative pressures within the third lumbar disk in various positions. Pressure is least while lying on the back and greatest while sitting forward. Pressure between disks is higher when sitting than when standing.

SOURCE: Reprinted with permission from *The Back Doctor*, by Hamilton Hall (New York: McGraw-Hill, 1980).

How to Have Sex

There are a number of pain-free ways: face-to-face, with both partners on their sides; or face-to-back, in what is sometimes called the "spoon" position, with the female nestled against the male's lap. There are, of course, many other possible positions, and the key to avoiding strain "is to make sure you do not arch your back or your neck" in any of them, says Dr. Hall.

How to Keep Fit

All sports involve some wear and tear on the spine. But that's no reason to sit on the sidelines, Dr. Hall says. "Apart from the trauma of an accident —which, after all, can happen anywhere to anybody—even the most vigorous sports activities won't harm your back; they may simply make it hurt for a few days." But "hurt is not the same as harm," Dr. Hall assures us, "and the

---

Miscellaneous Back Facts

Did you know that:

- High-heeled shoes are not a good idea because they cause you to arch your back more than normal. And even though much of the effect of high heels is dissipated through the ankles, knees, and hips by the time the spine is reached, the lift can be enough to cause pain that less lofty heels would not, particularly if your backache is a Type 1.

- If you're going to wear a back brace, do so as you would a pair of gloves—as something to be taken off when the job is done. "If a back brace gives you a feeling of abdominal support and confidence during certain activities, by all means wear it," Hamilton Hall, M.D., says. But take it off when that activity is over, "and try to strengthen your abdomen so that the brace becomes increasingly unnecessary," is Dr. Hall's advice.

- The force of gravity has a nasty effect on back problems: The families and doctors of U.S. astronauts aboard the 84-day voyage of Skylab in 1974 were more than a little surprised to find the spacemen nearly two inches taller upon their return. "With no gravity . . . their disks fattened up with moisture, making their

trade-off may be worth it to you, in immediate pleasure and in feeling like a normal person instead of a semi-invalid."

"Three forms of strain may be imposed upon your spine" by your fitness efforts, Dr. Hall says: "weight loading, rotation, and arching." Weight loading (which happens during weight lifting and jogging) tends to compress disks and cause facet joints to settle even more tightly together. Rotation (a common maneuver in squash, racquetball, tennis, and golf) can strain disks by tugging at the fibers of their outer shells. And arching (a common occurrence during hockey, basketball, baseball, rowing, canoeing, skiing, archery, and certain forms of swimming—especially the breaststroke) tends, like weight-loading sports, to create friction between facet joints.

Whatever you do for exercise, though, don't feel bad for learning to "cheat" in ways that minimize your discomforts. Hurt may not be harm. But it's not much fun, either.

---

spines longer and the men taller," Dr. Hall explains. "Once they returned to earth, gravity took over again, and within a few days the astronauts were back to normal size." Since that mission, space suits have been designed to allow for such growth.

- If you find that "cracking" your back (or neck) seems to help, go right ahead, Dr. Hall says. You could be performing a therapeutic release of tension, but you are not rearranging any bones. The sound you hear is the same as the one you hear when you crack your knuckles. "In the joints of your fingers and in your spinal joints you have nitrogen in solution, under pressure. If you pull suddenly on your finger, you decrease the pressure on the joint. This causes the nitrogen to come out of solution and turn temporarily from liquid to gas in much the same way that champagne goes 'pop' when you uncork the bottle." The noises a chiropractor can get out of you, unfortunately, are caused the same way. Chiropractic manipulation "can put your spine through a useful range of movements . . . and sometimes relieve muscle spasms," Dr. Hall says, "but any chiropractor who tells you he is actually changing the position of vertebrae in your spine is merely revealing his own ignorance of the way the back works." The disks of your back do not slip, and the facet joints do not keep "jumping out," Dr. Hall says. "Everything is already in place—there is nothing to 'put back.' "

39/

The Common Cold: Best Treated with Common Sense

What did you do for your last cold?

If you're like most Americans, you waited until it caused you considerable discomfort and then you fought it—with decongestants, antihistamines, and aspirin.

Too much, too late.

Cold remedies may soothe the symptoms of a cold, but they do nothing to speed its cure. Some, in fact, get in the way of your body's ability to cure itself.

And since more than 90 percent of us get between two and three colds a year (a blow to the economy of an estimated $6 billion in workdays that we either miss or muff), it's time we managed the common cold with common sense. Which is why we bring to you the following tales of Barbara and Bill.

Bill handled his cold badly; Barbara managed hers with wisdom and style. Barbara, as a result, missed about two hours of work. Bill blundered the better part of a week.

Feel free to identify with the story. And pay close attention to our footnotes at the end of it. They should give you the facts you need to keep your next cold a mild one—particularly if you're more of a Bill than a Barbara.

Bill still thinks he caught his cold at Saturday's football game.[1] He had worn only a sweater, and it rained from the third quarter on.

Actually, though, Bill's cold virus had been with him since Tuesday of the week before.[2] He picked it up by way of a handshake with a sales representative from Toledo.[3]

Bill complained of feeling a little "out of sorts" two days after that—Thursday night, as he sat down to supper—but he wrote the feeling off as being due to a hard day at the office. When he sneezed, he blamed it on his wife's heavy-handedness with the pepper.[4]

Friday morning found Bill a little slow to get out of bed. Once into it at work, though, he was "fine." That afternoon he did notice his throat feeling scratchy, but he attributed that to all the cigarette smoke at his boss's TGIF

office party.[5]

Buoyed by his drinks, Bill didn't make it home Friday until about 11:00 P.M. A short spat with his wife didn't help his night's sleep any, and so Saturday morning's ill feelings got dismissed as a combination of a bad night in bed and a slight hangover.

Bill's cold virus, at this point, had been given everything it needed to come down on him like a rock.

"Where's the aspirin?" was all Bill could say as he stood dripping wet inside the kitchen door following his Saturday afternoon soaking. He had chills. A headache. His joints ached. And the back of his throat felt like an emery board.[6]

But the aspirin made him feel better. And that night he and his wife kept their engagement with the Smiths.[7]

Sunday was Bill's big jogging day, and he was proud of not having missed it for over a year. The workout would "do him good," he told his wife. "Get rid of some of this stuffiness." (Bill's virus had begun its attack on the sensitive tissues lining his nose. And his body was responding by increasing blood flow and white blood cells to this area.[8])

But the run didn't help much. It cleared Bill up for a while, but by Sunday afternoon he could barely breathe.

"Do we have any cold pills?" was Bill's next request.

They did, unfortunately, and they made Bill's breathing a little easier. But they also cut off the supply of histamines to the injured tissues inside Bill's nose. And it was these histamines that were promoting the blood flow—and hence inflammation—that Bill's nose needed to repair itself. Bill remarked to his wife what a marvelous "cure" he thought cold pills were before going on to spend the entire second half of the Dallas vs. Pittsburgh football game in a drug-induced slumber.[9]

Monday, of course, meant off to work as usual. After all, Bill "only had a cold." And he had "an important meeting," besides.

That meeting went as poorly as the rest of Bill's week: He banged up the car Monday night on the way to his Lion's Club meeting; he fell asleep Tuesday afternoon during a crucial sales presentation; he received a "get on the stick" memo from his boss on Wednesday; and on Thursday he missed his plane flight to Toledo. If only he had listened to his body—like Barbara did.

Barbara works with Bill. And she also shook hands with the sales rep from Toledo on Tuesday. But when she felt "out of sorts" two days later, she did something about it.

First of all, she took a full gram (1,000 milligrams) of vitamin C.[10] Then she drew herself a warm bath and took almost an hour to decide what she was *not* going to do the next day:

- She was *not* going to feel obligated to get to work on time, and if she went to work at all, she was going to catch up on some light paperwork. Her afternoon appointment in New York would have to wait.[11]

- She was *not* going to take any cold remedies. If her cold was going to be a bad one, she wanted to know about it—and rest accordingly.
- She was going to drink a lot of fluids, to compensate for her virus's drying effect on the tissues of her nose and throat—but she was *not* going to make them (as Bill had) cocktails.[12]
- She was going to switch from coffee to herb tea for a day to help her body slow down and get the rest it needed to fight her infection.
- She was going to stop smoking to keep from further irritating the already parched tissues of her throat.
- She was going to simplify her diet (more soups, fruits, and vegetables; less greasy foods and sweets) so as not to tax her system with a lot of heavy-duty digestion.

When Barbara's husband called her for dinner, she felt better already. She had chicken soup and some fresh fruit, read for a while, went to bed at 9:30 with her electric blanket on medium, and made it to work on Friday in time to be invited—by Bill—to have a drink over lunch.

"No, thanks, Bill. I think I may be coming down with a cold. Think I'll just have a cup of soup and a glass of juice."

"Guess you won't be making the office party, then."

"Probably not."

She didn't. And felt well enough to enjoy the Dallas vs. Pittsburgh football game—in person—by Sunday.

Footnotes Worth Noting

1. Colds are not caused by getting a chill. They are caused by any one of an estimated two hundred different viruses (which is one reason why a cure for the common cold may be a long way off). Getting chilled, however, can serve as a catalyst capable of bringing viruses to life. "It is not the chilling itself which causes the infection," says Hal Zina Bennett in *Cold Comfort* (Clarkson N. Potter, 1980), but rather "the chilling encourages viruses already present to multiply and, at the same time, set up an environment relatively free of antibodies that might otherwise discourage the virus."
2. Most cold viruses undergo a one-to-six-day period of incubation before causing any noticeable symptoms.

3. Colds are spread more effectively by direct contact—such as handshakes and kisses—than they are by sneezes and coughs. And they are most contagious in their early stages—a day or so before symptoms may even be noticed.

4. The first noticeable signs of a cold are apt to be very subtle ones: a slight tickle in the throat, a feeling of tightness and/or dryness in the nose, feelings of being generally out of sorts (mildly distracted, physically uncoordinated, tense), appetite not up to par.

5. "The process the body goes through to heal a cold or flu requires about the same energy as hard physical labor," Bennett reports. Hence, feelings of fatigue as the body works to restore cells damaged by the attacking virus. One of the most noticeable effects of this tissue damage may be a scratchy throat, caused in part by substances the body produces to counteract viral invasions.

6. Aches and pains of the joints and head are natural consequences of running a slight fever, which is what Bill's body was doing in an attempt to fight his infection. Higher temperatures reduce the rate of virus reproduction.

7. Aspirin should be used with caution to relieve cold discomforts because they can make you feel better than you are.

8. Any vigorous exercise should be avoided during the early stages of a cold. If you must exercise, do just enough to improve your mood.

9. Inflammation is a necessary evil in the healing process.

10. Vitamin C's effects on cold viruses are still being studied. Enough information exists, however, for us to suggest taking one to three grams a day at the outset of a cold, and daily doses of at least 500 milligrams throughout its duration. Daily supplements of up to 500 milligrams—year round—are also a good idea.

11. Stress has been shown to impose specific strains on the body, not the least of which (as far as colds are concerned) are: reduced blood flow, reduced moisture, and reduced antibody production in the areas of the nasal passages and mouth.

12. Alcohol can make us feel no pain—a dangerous situation when the secret to curing a cold is feeling and responding to as many pains as possible. As Bennett puts it: "The most healthy response to the pain and discomfort of the healing phase of a cold or flu is to acknowledge the discomfort as your body's call for cooperation in the healing process."

Amen.

40/

Halitosis—Yesterday and Today

You can be fit as a fiddle, neat as a pin, smart as a whip, and about the nicest person around. But if you've got bad breath, you've got problems.

A silly modern-day hang-up of ours? History doesn't seem to think so.

The King of Wales decreed back in the tenth century that any woman who left home within the first seven years of marriage could make no claims on her husband's property unless at least one of her reasons for leaving was a good one. Impotence and halitosis were considered two.

And when King Henry VII several centuries later sent envoys to assess the suitability of the widowed Queen of Naples as a marriage partner, he instructed them "to mark her breasts . . . whether they be big or small," and "to approach as near to her mouth as they honestly may to the intent of feeling its condition."

Bad breath is—and always has been—high on our list of turnoffs.

What causes it?

A number of things: unhealthy gums, dirty teeth, poor digestion, a pasty tongue, a dry mouth, savory spices, alcohol, tobacco, and—believe it or not— mouthwash. Let's look at the most common of these culprits first.

Unhealthy gums. Michael Lerner, D.M.D., a dentist from Lexington, Kentucky, says that inflamed or infected gums affect about 95 percent of us, which translates into varying degrees of halitosis *for 95 percent of us, too,* because we're "blowing air over something that doesn't smell good."

Dr. Lerner says gum inflammation develops when bacteria accumulate on the teeth and produce toxic waste products that irritate and weaken gum tissue. These sites of inflammation are not always visible to the eye, he warns, but if your gums bleed when you brush your teeth, it means you've got them.

The problem in most cases, though, is easy to correct. Two or three days of proper brushing and flossing, Dr. Lerner says, will "disrupt the bacteria and increase tissue resistance." He also recommends taking "good levels" of vitamins A and C, and getting plenty of bioflavonoids (prevalent in the pulps and rinds of fruit).

Dirty teeth. Whether or not there are (as seventeenth-century scientist Anton van Leeuwenhoek maintained) "more animals living in the scum on a man's teeth than there are men in a whole kingdom," teeth *can* get bacterially busy. Brushing after every meal (with or without toothpaste) or swishing the mouth well with water (if brushing is awkward) can remove food debris on which these bacteria feed.

A filmy tongue.   Inflamed gums may be the most popular cause of bad breath, but according to an experiment done recently by Joseph Tonzevitch, Ph.D., a professor in the School of Dentistry at the University of British Columbia, a foul tongue may be the most potent.

Dr. Tonzevitch asked eight victims of "morning mouth" to use one of three methods to allay this common affliction: brushing the teeth, brushing the tongue, or brushing both. Before and after each of these scrubbings, Dr. Tonzevitch measured the amount of odor (in the form of sulphur-containing gases) expelled in some sample exhalations. His findings:

- Brushing just the teeth reduced odor by 25 percent.
- Brushing just the tongue reduced odor by 75 percent.
- Brushing both brought about a reduction in oral stench of 85 percent.

Dr. Tonzevitch's conclusion: "Tongue brushing is the single most effective method of decreasing breath odor." (The Romans did it, and Muhammad is reported to have encouraged his followers to obey the practice, also.) Use a soft-bristle toothbrush, go lightly, and don't feel as though you have to use toothpaste.

Inadequate digestion.   Brushing our teeth and our tongues, then, can reduce breath odors by 85 percent. Where's the rest coming from?

Inside our bodies, Dr. Tonzevitch says. "Chemicals produced by the metabolic activities of the body, such as digestion, are picked up in the blood and eliminated through the lungs via the mouth."

Can these foul winds from within be freshened?

Maybe. If your problem is a shortage of digestive enzymes (which is preventing food in your stomach from being completely digested), you are not in as much luck as folks who are simply overindulging in the wrong foods: white flour, refined sugar, and caffeine, says Bruce Pacetti, D.D.S., the director of nutritional research at Florida Holistic Medical Center in Clearwater. "These foods can upset human biochemistry, which can result in either the fermentation of carbohydrates or the putrefaction of proteins in the digestive tract."

Tobacco.   One English health publication has likened smoker's breath to "the musty smell that lingers in the damp basements of secondhand bookstores." (If you are well read enough to recognize that as being true, congratulations.) Dampness, however, is just the opposite of a smoker's problem; *dryness* is what's forcing his breath afoul, in addition to the smell of tobacco. "Runner's breath" (due to thirst after a hard workout) and "cotton mouth" (due to thirst after a hard night) are two other instances of breath dropping below par due to dehydration.

Alcohol.   Alcohol may sweeten breath initially, but by robbing the body of water, alcohol's ultimate contributions are not aromatic ones.

Mouthwash.   Like alcohol, mouthwashes may tidy things up for a while (several hours at best), but the end result of repeated dousings with astringents is bad. "Mouthwash is terrible," Philip Parsons, D.D.S., a dentist from Keystone Heights, Florida, told us. "It lowers bacteria for an hour or two, but more grow back than before."

What's more, if the alcohol in mouthwash (Astring-O-Sol is 140 proof) is used daily, it can begin to damage tissue in the mouth and throat—causing the very sort of inflammations your breath would be better off without.

So what's a foul mouth to do?

- Brush the teeth—and tongue—at least twice a day.
- Avoid excess sugar, white flour, and caffeine.
- Go easy on alcohol.
- And regard smoking as a one-way ticket to loneliness.

41/

Bad Skin: Tips for Giving Your Mug Its Best Shot

If a picture is worth a thousand words, your face is worth a million. Because it's an incorrigible tattletale. And it always tells the truth.

"It's the mirror of what goes on inside us, emotionally as well as physically," one dermatologist has said. Leave it to your face to broadcast a big night out on the town as vividly as a half-hour run.

Why?

Because your face is the most visible part of the largest organ of your body: your skin.

"The skin of an average adult weighs more than twice as much as the brain or heart and it's far more active than many people realize," writes dermatologist Irwin I. Lubowe, M.D., in *New Hope for Your Skin* (Pocket, 1966). Each square inch contains: 78 nerves, 650 sweat glands, 19 or 20 blood vessels, 78 sensory mechanisms for heat, 13 sensory mechanisms for cold, 1,300 nerve endings for recording pain, 160 to 165 pressure points for the sense of touch, 95 to 100 sebaceous glands, 65 hairs and muscles, and about 19,500 cells.

Spread this complex arrangement over 21 square feet of arms, legs, torso, and head, and you're looking at a *very* influential organ. In addition to holding you together, your skin:

- protects you from germs,
- warms you,
- cools you,
- excretes harmful toxins,
- takes in oxygen,
- gives off carbon dioxide,
- and secretes its own moisturizers.

Your skin, in other words, is hardly a helpless coating. It can take care of itself *in addition* to taking care of you. But . . .

It needs to be fed. Not fussed with from the outside, but nourished—from the *inside*.

"Nutrition for the skin is just like that for any other part of the body," says Dr. Lubowe. "It comes from the bloodstream, not the surface. Skin needs proteins to manufacture new cells, carbohydrates for energy, and certain vitamins and minerals for specialized purposes."

Skin also, believe it or not, needs exercise. Because exercise steps up blood flow, and increased blood flow provides skin cells with more of the nutrients —and oxygen—that they need to stay healthy. An experiment done several years ago with a group of men in Finland bears this out.

When compared with samples taken from 29 sedentary men of similar ages (31 to 68), skin samples taken from 29 very active men (who were daily runners and/or cross-country skiers) showed greater elasticity and thickness— two very important weapons in the fight against facial wrinkles caused by aging. (Wrinkling is the result of cell degeneration and the breakdown of an elastic

What to Feed Your Face

The skin, like other organs, requires proper nutrition supplied by a balanced diet. And, "since nourishment for the skin comes from the bloodstream, not the surface, the idea of feeding the skin from the outside makes about as much sense as trying to heat a stove by rubbing its outer surfaces." These words come from Irwin I. Lubowe, M.D.

It is more important to eat right, in other words, than to anoint. Fresh fruits and vegetables for vitamins A and C; low-fat dairy products and fish for vitamin D, essential fatty acids, and protein; whole grain cereals, beans, and whole grain breads for B vitamins and vitamin E. To perform all its daily functions properly, your skin needs all of the above —particularly as you get older.

"In older people, there is usually poor absorption and slow metabolism," Dr. Lubowe says. "For all my patients over 50 who have skin disorders, I routinely suggest 25,000 units of vitamin A per day, 500 milligrams of vitamin C, and an all-purpose vitamin and mineral capsule. These are the vitamins needed for production and maintenance of skin integrity in the aging."

A word on weight. Dr. Lubowe says that, "As far as the skin is concerned, heavy people are prone to have more trouble than people of normal weight, partly because they chafe themselves where skin gathers in folds, partly because they perspire more than those of lighter build, and partly because the circulatory system must do much more work to serve the excess poundage" (*The Modern Guide to Skin Care and Beauty*, E. P. Dutton, 1973).

skin component called collagen—both of which appear to be retarded by habitual aerobic exercise.)

Skin responds to exercise by strengthening its structure and increasing its mass, possibly because "many of the functions of the skin itself get subjected to dramatic metabolic changes during exercise," the researchers said.

Your skin, in other words, works right along with the rest of you as your exercise. It sweats, excretes toxins, turns over fresh supplies of nutrients and oxygen. And so as your muscles, heart, and lungs get in shape, so does your hide.

Which may be why the nonexercisers in your office look so pasty. And the joggers glow. (My wife, instead of putting on makeup, now goes for a two-mile run when she wants to look her best.)

What else can you do for your face? You can:

- *Go easy on scrubbing it with soap.* Except for skin that is excessively oily, most dermatologists recommend simply a washcloth and warm—not hot—water.
- *Avoid getting sunburned.* Lightly bronzed is one thing, but broiled is another. More than a couple of hours a week of direct sunlight can increase your chances of getting skin cancer and also contribute to facial wrinkling. If you *are* out in the sun a lot, use a sunscreen (*not* a tanning lotion). Or wear a wide-brimmed hat. Approach sunlamps and tanning parlors sensibly, too.
- *Don't smoke.* Smoking, by constricting blood vessels, impairs circulation. And impaired circulation means premature wrinkling, as a California study several years ago showed dramatically. Harry W. Daniell, M.D., studied 1,104 people for "crow's-feet" and found that "smokers in the 40- to 49-year age group were as likely to be prominently wrinkled as nonsmokers who were 20 years older." He also found the complexions among smokers to be of a decidedly "yellow-gray pallor." So starved for blood were their faces, in fact, that Dr. Daniell noticed many had lost the ability to blush (*Annals of Internal Medicine*, December, 1971).
- *Don't overdrink.* Excessive drinking can dilate facial blood vessels —permanently. What's behind a red nose is a matrix of broken veins.
- *If you must lose weight, do it slowly.* Crash diets can leave your skin wondering where you went. Gradual weight loss, on the other hand, gives your exterior a chance to follow along.
- *Try not to squint.* Squinting puts out a welcome mat for crow's-feet. Get yourself a pair of eyeglasses and/or sunglasses, instead.
- *Keep your house well humidified,* particularly during the winter. Dry skin is the first step to wrinkled skin.

- *If you must lubricate your skin,* use a natural vegetable oil like sesame, olive, peanut, safflower, or avocado. They're every bit as good as commercial products, and they're a far-sight cheaper.

How much can all this really change the way you look?

Maybe a lot, considering how much the way you look is affected by the way you feel.

As the Roman philosopher Publilius Syrus said over two thousand years ago, "A fair exterior is a silent recommendation." It shows that the person inside is feeling good about making the most of what he's got.

Beauty goes more than skin deep.

42/
Looking for Dr. Right

Wouldn't we all love a Marcus Welby—a proven professional willing to come to our homes and have coffee with us in our times of need . . . an M.D., psychiatrist, marriage counselor, and priest all wrapped up into one? What's a member of the Marcus Welby fan club to do?

Get looking.

There *are* good doctors out there. The problem is that we, as patients, aren't taking the time to find them.

If you're into fitness and feeling invincible because of it, you may not care that your doctor is a robot. Or that he's been treating *you* like one.

But go on the blink—as all of us can—and you may find yourself regretting that relationship. When faced with a serious medical decision, you want to be able to consult not just someone who knows your body, but someone who knows *you*. The personality factor, most doctors agree, is a very important ingredient in the healing process.

"The placebo effect can be very strong in the field of personal health care," says Hal Strelnick, M.D., a family practitioner on the editorial board of the Health Policy Advisory Center in New York City. "If you believe in and trust a treatment, it's more apt to work."

And the relationship between doctor and patient is important for more than just psychological reasons, Dr. Strelnick says. "You're more apt to follow a doctor's orders when you feel that time and care have gone into your diagnosis." When compliance is hard medicine to swallow, in other words, trust can do a lot to improve its flavor.

So, how do you go about finding this true-blue doctor of your dreams?

Step one is to decide what—if anything—is wrong with the physician you've got. (Maybe it's *you* that's to blame for your rotten relationship. Are you secretive? Irked by the cost of health care in general? That's not your doctor's fault.)

Step two is to decide what sort of person might be an improvement on what you've already got. Might it be an older doctor with more experience? Someone younger and more familiar with the latest philosophies and techniques? Or maybe you want a doctor of the same sex.

Once you've gotten these basics out of the way, it's out you go—shopping. And the best way to do that, Dr. Strelnick says, is "word of mouth." Start with close friends, then move on to neighbors, relatives, and people with whom you work.

Beware of horror stories, though, Dr. Strelnick warns. "If someone tells you he wouldn't go to a certain so-and-so if you paid him, it could be because the doctor asked him to do something he didn't want to—like quit smoking." Get to the bottom of all reports, fair or foul, that you receive.

If relocation is the reason you're in search of a new doc, ask your current one for some help. "He may have an old med school buddy, someone he respects, in practice in your new hometown," say Keith W. Sehnert, M.D., and Howard Eisenberg in their book *How to Be Your Own Doctor—Sometimes* (Grosset and Dunlap, 1975). "He may be willing to phone an acquaintance— a former nurse, a hospital administrator, an officer in the county medical society —to solicit off-the-record recommendations."

You can check the credentials of a doctor for yourself by consulting the *American Medical Directory* and the *Directory of Medical Specialists*, available in some public and most medical libraries. They'll tell you where a doctor went to medical school, his specialty, and whether or not he is certified by the American Specialty Board. (Board certification means the doctor has completed a three- to seven-year training program and passed a series of competency exams in his specialty.)

Once you've hit on a prospect that sounds strong, the next step is to schedule an appointment to meet him or her in person. You should expect to pay for it, of course, as you would any office visit—but considering it's going to be *you* this time doing the examining, it stands to be an expense well invested. Here are some things to look for:

- "He or she should be a warm person who gives the impression of liking his work," says Dale Dodson, D.O., past president of the American Osteopathic Association. "And he should have the integrity to tell you when he doesn't know an answer."
- "I look for someone who will treat me with respect," says Joseph Nowell, executive director of the International Academy of Preventive Medicine. "I also don't want a physician who just says, 'Okay, here's your prescription.' If I'm having headaches, I want to know why."
- Take notice of the office atmosphere, suggests Merle Hoffman, founder and director of CHOICES, a comprehensive ambulatory health care facility in New York City. Is it genuinely friendly? Or cold and calculating?

Be the aggressor in this first meeting. Ask about controversial subjects. Does this doctor advocate vitamins? How important is good nutrition? Exercise? How has he chosen to conduct his own life in these areas?

If the doctor is any good, he'll take the time to open up to you, even if it means inviting you to call him back by phone sometime when he's not busy. "Any doctor who won't come to the phone when he isn't busy isn't worth seeing—and that goes for specialists, too," says Alan L. Goldberg, M.D., former president of the New York State Academy of Family Physicians.

If you find yourself coming away from this first meeting with serious doubts, see the writing on the wall. If you can't agree on things even when there's nothing at stake, what might your chances be of accepting a recommendation somewhere down the line that you undergo radical surgery? Not good.

Ms. Hoffman, an advocate of "patient power," feels that we as medical consumers have been conditioned to be passive. And that it's time we take a more active role in making decisions about our health. We're more educated than we've ever been.

And after all . . . who really knows more about the way you feel than you do?

PART IV/
ANSWERS TO QUESTIONS PLEASURE SEEKERS ASK MOST

Preventive Medicine to the Rescue

We have a question and answer section in the *Executive Fitness Newsletter* that has taught me a great deal about health. It's taught me that Dan Zeismiller can break out in a rash whenever his golf score exceeds 100; that Sue Ann Warner's left knee doesn't like to run more than about 14 miles a week; that Carl Smith can lose weight but not his lovehandles.

What I've learned from that question and answer section, quite simply, is that health is an amazingly individual affair. So individual, in fact, that the medical profession seems to be having some problems with it. Why else would all these questions be coming to us?

We've even had questions from M.D.'s themselves. Which is very flattering, but it's also a little distressing. Because what it suggests is that the kind of medical information people—even doctors—now want is in short supply.

And what kind of information is that?

Information on health rather than disease. The medical profession, by devoting its energies to fixing us once we're sick, has fallen behind in being able to coach us on how to stay well.

Health information, however, is out there. It's just that you have to know where to look for it. In answering the following questions (which I consider to be some of the more interesting and relevant that the *Executive Fitness Newsletter* has received over the past four years), we had to consult sports medicine specialists, nutritionists, physiologists, psychologists, and M.D.'s considered slightly renegade by their peers. Together, these folks comprise an up-and-coming new field called preventive medicine. They don't have *all* the answers, of course; no one does. But I think you'll agree the answers they do have are pretty interesting.

43/
Questions and Answers

Q/ How many calories do I burn playing 18 holes of golf?

A/ That depends on how big you are, how bad you are, and how you get from green to green. We'll base our calculations on the following assumptions: first, that you weigh in the neighborhood of 180 pounds; second, that you do not stray too "bogishly" from the fairways; and third, that you either pull or carry your clubs. (If you drive a cart, you're not getting much more exercise than driving your car.)

Most clubs weigh about 20 pounds. And the average 18-hole course covers about 6,175 yards, roughly 3½ miles. We're going to figure that you actually walk close to four, though, because the distance between tees—and the amount you "stray"—must be considered.

Feeding all this into our computer, and basing our calculations on a walking speed that would get you around an 18-hole course in about four hours (one mile per hour), we came up with a grand total of 1,540 calories. If you pull your clubs, figure slightly less. And for you ladies, assuming you weigh in the neighborhood of 120 pounds, your grand total of expended calories comes to about 1,000.

Each 12-ounce celebrational beer back at the club house, incidentally, is good for about 150 calories. You might want to "keep score" with that in mind.

Q/ Why does my skin get dry every winter and what can I do about it?

A/ Many winter-related dry skin conditions are due to shortages of vitamins A and D—vitamin A because we tend to eat fewer fresh vegetables during the winter, and vitamin D because we tend also to get less sunshine. (Vitamin D is produced when the skin is exposed to sunlight, an infrequent event during the short, cold days of winter.)

Vitamin A's role is to help skin replenish itself on a cellular level, from the inside out, and vitamin D's job is to help the skin use calcium, "a great 201 quieter of skin problems," says Carl Reich, M.D. (Dr. Reich has been treating cold-weather skin problems where it's *really* cold—in Alberta, Canada.)

The solution for these deficiencies?

Either more vegetables and sunshine . . . or fish liver oil.

"I have dry skin in the winter," Gerald Green, another Canadian M.D., told us, "particularly on the back of my hands and on my feet. But three times a day I take a halibut liver oil capsule that contains 5,000 I.U. of vitamin A and 400 I.U. of vitamin D and that keeps the problem in check quite well." Cod-liver oil also comes highly recommended.

Dr. Green credits the moistening effects of fish liver oils to more than just vitamins, however. Fish oils add extra *oil* to the system, he told us, which has a lubricating effect on the skin.

Fewer baths (especially hot ones) and less soap (particularly the deodorizing kind) can also help dry skin. Jonathan Zizmor, M.D. (co-author of *Super Skin*, Thomas Y. Crowell, 1976), recommends washing with imitation soaps or—if you're really dry—no soap at all.

And, of course, covering hands and face from Old Man Winter's drying winds will also help keep your skin moist.

Q/ Does it make much difference how fast I run for burning calories?

A/ No. The more important consideration is how *far* you run. "Pace has very little effect on the caloric cost of running, and thus individuals in low fitness

Calories Used per Mile of Running

Weight (pounds)	Rate of Running (pace per mile)								
	5:20	6:00	6:40	7:20	8:00	8:40	9:20	10:00	10:40
120	83	83	81	80	79	78	77	76	75
130	90	89	88	87	85	84	83	82	81
140	97	95	94	93	92	91	89	88	87
150	103	102	101	99	98	97	95	94	93
160	110	109	107	106	104	103	101	100	99
170	117	115	113	112	111	109	107	106	105
180	123	121	120	119	117	115	114	112	111
190	130	128	127	125	123	121	120	118	117
200	137	135	133	131	129	128	126	124	123
210	143	141	139	137	136	134	132	130	129
220	150	148	146	144	142	140	138	136	135

NOTE: Expenditure of 3,500 calories equals one pound of weight loss.

SOURCE: Reprinted from *The New Guide to Distance Running* by the editors of *Runner's World*. Copyright 1978 by World Publications, Mountain View, Calif. Used with permission.

categories can expend almost as much energy as a similarly sized, conditioned person for a given distance," reported a team of doctors several years ago in the *Journal of the American Medical Association* (April 22, 1974). The accompanying table should make that quite clear.

What *does* make a difference, however, is body weight, as you can see. A nimble 120-pounder burns up only 83 calories per mile at a 5:20 clip, whereas a lusty 220-pounder expends nearly twice that.

Inspired?

Q/ Should sex be curtailed following a heart attack?

A/ Not if it's with someone you're used to. The anxiety, not to mention the exercise, of taking on someone new could be more than you're up to, but sex with somebody "familiar," most authorities agree, may be resumed usually within three to eight weeks of a myocardial infarction.

Studies have shown that having sex with a spouse is about as strenuous as briskly climbing a flight of stairs; so if you can make it to the bedroom, chances are you'll be fine.

To play it safe, however, Joseph S. Alpert, M.D., author of *The Heart Attack Hand Book* (Little, Brown, 1978), recommends certain precautions. Avoid having sex, he says:

- immediately after a large meal,
- for three hours after drinking alcohol,
- in extremely hot or cold temperatures,
- before or after strenuous activity,
- if you are feeling anger or resentment,
- or when you are very fatigued.

It is also a good idea, Dr. Alpert says, to allow ample time for "warm-up," meaning foreplay, and to consider, too, the possibility of being intimate the first few times without actually reaching a point of climax.

Things to watch out for are rapid heart rate and/or heavy breathing that lasts 20 to 30 minutes after sex, chest pain during or after intercourse, or sleeplessness or extreme fatigue on the day following an encounter. These could be signs that your rehabilitation is being rushed. Take your time. The rate of total sexual recovery from most heart attacks is very good.

Q/ Is smoking marijuana as bad for the lungs as smoking cigarettes?

A/ It looks as though it may be worse. And for several reasons.

First, people tend to inhale marijuana smoke more deeply, and hold these inhalations longer. This gives the toxic elements in marijuana smoke greater exposure to sensitive lung tissue.

Then, there's the matter of these toxic elements themselves. And from what researchers have been able to determine, they appear to be of equal mutagenic (potentially cancer-causing) activity as those in tobacco.

Add to this the fact that the *amount* of these impurities has been estimated to be far greater in marijuana smoke than in smoke from cigarettes, and the prognosis for a high and healthy life looks dimmer still. According to research done recently at the University of California School of Public Health in Berkeley, the amount of tar contained in one marijuana cigarette is equal to that of 1½ high-tar cigarettes, or 100 (that's *five packs*) low-tar cigarettes made from tobacco.

What specific effects can these tar levels have on lung function?

Not good, particularly when pot is smoked daily and for long periods of time. Donald Tashkin, M.D., a pulmonary specialist from the University of California at Los Angeles, found that marijuana smokers who smoked an average of five joints a week for at least two years had poorer lung function than a group of computer-matched tobacco smokers good for 16 or more cigarettes a day

Q/ How good are the mini-trampolines for exercise?

A/ Finally, we have some reliable data to answer that question. And the answer is "quite good, indeed."

That assessment comes from James White, Ph.D. Dr. White, director of human performance and sports medicine at the University of California at San Diego and author of *Jump for Joy* (University of California at San Diego Press, 1981), has recently completed an extensive series of tests on rebound exercisers.

"In perhaps our most convincing [series of tests]," Dr. White told us, "we took 70 overweight women, put 20 on an exercise program involving running on a treadmill, 20 on stationary bicycles, 20 on mini-trampolines, and 10 doing nothing. The programs were identical in that each involved 10 minutes of warm-up exercises, followed by 30 minutes of work on the respective devices, followed by 10 minutes of cool-down. The 30 minutes were conducted at 80 to 85 percent of the women's maximum heart rates."

The results?

"After ten weeks, all three of the exercise groups showed significant— and *equivalent*—gains, leading us to conclude that the jumping devices were *as* good as, and in some ways *better* than, running or cycling."

Why better?

"Because with the jumping devices, fewer women sustained injuries. Whereas 50 percent of the runners came down with some sort of leg problems, and some of the cyclists complained of calf strain, none of the jumpers were bothered by any pains whatsoever."

Then, too, Dr. White said, there was the all-important matter of sticking to it. "When we followed up on each of those groups a year later, we found that only 5 percent of the cyclists were still at it, 31 percent of the joggers had kept up, but a surprising 58 percent of the jumpers had continued with their programs. And we had similar results with a group of 185 executives we tested. After a two-year period, we found that 78 percent of the women and 52 percent of the men were still jumping."

Q/ How dangerous is it to breathe smoke from other people's cigarettes?

A/ That depends on several factors: the concentration of the smoke you are exposed to, the frequency of your exposures, how much of the smoke you are being exposed to has already been inhaled, and how healthy you are.

According to Ruth Winter, author of *The Scientific Case Against Smoking* (Crown Publishers, 1980), when a filtered cigarette is smoked, its smoker inhales only about 23 percent of the smoke the cigarette produces. And of this 23 percent, about 30 percent gets exhaled. So when a smoker lights up, he in one way or another offers those around him a generous 84 percent of his habit—enough under some conditions to raise blood nicotine levels of nonsmoking bystanders to as much as 20 percent of his own.

F. Schmidt, M.D., author of "Health Risks of Passive Smoking" (*World Smoking and Health*, Spring, 1978), says that a cigarette capable of producing 30 milligrams of tar can render the air in an enclosed room "unhealthy" according to air quality index standards specified by the U.S. Environmental Protection Agency. Eye and throat irritation, lung impairment, worsening of existing respiratory and circulatory ills, and decreased exercise performance are among the health hazards secondhand smoke exposures can impose.

The reason that secondhand (sidestream) smoke is so toxic is that it's unfiltered. The smoke that comes *off* a cigarette can contain three times as much tar and ten times greater concentrations of cancer-causing agents as the smoke that goes *through* it. James R. White, Ph.D., and Herman F. Froeb, M.D., report that chronic exposures to the tobacco smoke of others can result in lung damage equal to that suffered by smokers good for one to ten cigarettes a day. If you can smell it all day, chances are you're being affected, Dr. White says. And cigar smoke may be even worse. The gaseous and particulate compounds in cigars are found in concentrations which equal or exceed those found in cigarettes.

Pipes? American Lung Association spokesperson William Anderson, M.D., puts them in the same league as cigars.

Q/ Can smoking affect a man's sex drive?

A/ Yes, but for what reasons doctors aren't yet exactly sure.

In two studies recently completed in France, researchers H. Cendron and J. Vallery-Masson found that men between the ages of 25 and 40 who smoked one or more packs a day showed a greater decline in sexual activity than nonsmokers of the same age. And Paul S. Larson, Ph.D., at the University of Virginia, has found that impotence seems to be more prevalent among servicemen who are heavy smokers.

Brian Mattes, an officer of Smok-Enders in New Jersey, thinks it's simply a matter of fitness. "People who don't smoke, or who have quit, are in better shape. The oxygen level in their blood is higher, their body chemistries are free of poisons. Then, too, they smell better."

Not all explanations, however, are so simple. Dr. M. H. Briggs, a physician from Australia, theorizes that smoking cigarettes produces carbon monoxide in the blood, which in turn inhibits the production of the male sex hormone testosterone. He cites a comparative study of smokers and nonsmokers matched for height, weight, and marital status in which testosterone levels for the nonsmokers averaged a healthy 7.47 nanograms per milliliter of blood. Men who smoked 30 or more cigarettes a day could muster no better than an average of 5.15. What's more, the testosterone levels of the smokers bounced back to near normal in just seven days after they quit.

Smoking also seems to affect fertility. Carl Schirren, M.D., of the University of Hamburg in Germany, has reported cases of "severe disturbances of sperm motility" in men who smoked between 20 and 40 cigarettes a day. And in a study involving 3,605 hamsters, cited by the medical journal *Toxicology* back in 1973 (vol. I), heavy doses of nicotine were responsible for an actual shrinking of the sex organs themselves.

There is even evidence to suggest that men who smoke heavily may increase their chances of fathering stillborn, premature, or in some way malformed children.

Admittedly, many smoking studies rely on questionnaires and as a result have come under considerable criticism for being less than airtight. A testimony by one 82-year-old doctor who has been a specialist on smoking for 59 years, however, would seem hard to debunk. "I have seen literally thousands of quitters say they feel more energetic, healthy, and alive, many of whom will confess only as an afterthought that their sex lives have improved since they've quit. . . . And that you really can't know the difference until you've tried."

Q/ Can regular exercise help prevent cancer?

A/ We wish we could say yes. But until scientists better understand the disease, we'll have to restrict ourselves to reporting the encouraging results of two studies—and say maybe.

In one, Dennis Colacino, Ph.D., and Dr. Bruno Balke of the Department of Physical Education at the University of Wisconsin compared the growth rates of cancerous tumors in two groups of mice. One group was made to run a treadmill for 20 minutes a day, while the other group was kept inactive. After 17 weeks, tumor growth was twice as great in the inactive group.

Looking at humans, Dr. Ernst van Aaken of Germany compared cancer rates among 454 physically active men (between the ages of 40 and 89) with a similar group of sedentaries. He found the disease to be six times more prevalent in the inactive group.

Possible explanations?

Theories vary. Dr. van Aaken proposes that exercise keeps cells resistant to cancer by keeping them well supplied with oxygen. Others feel increased nutrient uptake and improved blood flow may be at play.

Q/ Is it bad to skip lunch?

A/ That depends on lunch, and also on what you had for breakfast. If lunch is normally an eight or nine hundred calorie affair that includes a cocktail, by all means, skip it. Prepare for this "fast," however, by eating a substantial breakfast—one containing at least a third of your daily need for protein.

If, on the other hand, you find that skipping lunch leaves you weak and headachy, try an eight-ounce container of yogurt, or some fresh fruit, or a small salad, or even just a piece of cheese to remind your stomach that you haven't abandoned it entirely.

There is probably no danger, however, in skipping meals. Studies with rats have shown that those whose diets are restricted invariably live longer than rats who are allowed to eat all they want. It might actually be healthier to go around feeling hungrier than we do.

Perhaps the most spartan—and slimming—substitute for lunch is exercise. Twenty or 30 minutes of vigorous exercise, if you're already reasonably fit, mobilizes glycogen (a form of blood sugar stored in your muscles and liver) with the result being a feeling of renewed energy very similar to that afforded by food. Depending on your degree of fitness, this feeling can last for several hours.

If you do skip lunch, however, don't fall prey to the "now I can stuff myself" syndrome at night. A triple-decker ham and cheese sandwich is better eaten at noon than at midnight.

Q/ Should a woman exercise during painful menstruation?

A/ Yes. Exercise can ease the discomforts. According to a recent report from the President's Council on Fitness, 70 to 80 percent of the women who suffer dysmenorrhea are guilty of poor living habits—with bad posture and lack of exercise leading the list. Irritability and tension also tend to heighten menstrual ills, so exercise, with its potential for being as good for the spirits as it is for the spine would seem the ideal medicine.

Are some activities more medicinal than others? Not really. Anything that exercises the major muscle groups and gets you breathing is good for cramps. Jogging, swimming, cycling. There's no reason to discontinue anything, actually, that you may be doing regularly.

As for specific exercises, giving your lower stomach a good heavy-handed massage can help. As can stretching for the hips and lower back. Sit-ups, too, are good. Eight weeks of the bent-knee variety done on a daily basis were found to make life a lot easier once a month for 36 college women tested by a team of doctors recently.

Midol, move over. When it comes to dispelling the ill humors of menstruation, good old-fashioned exercise is tough to beat.

Q/ What causes puffy eyes?

A/ Fluid can collect around—and under—the eyes for various reasons. Thomas O. Burkholder, M.D., an ophthalmologist from Allentown, Pennsylvania, points out that keeping the head in a "dependent" position (meaning level with or below the heart) can cause tissue around the eyes to swell. Anytime blood has to move "uphill" to get back to the heart, he explains, there is an increased tendency for swelling (hence the age-old recommendation to keep a sprained ankle elevated). Sleeping, working hunched over at your desk, scrubbing floors—all put the eyes under or at least level with the heart. Puffiness can result, particularly as we get older.

"Skin tends to lose its elasticity as we age," Dr. Burkholder says, and so the tissue around the eyes becomes all the more susceptible to "tugs" from swelling or just plain old gravity. Fatigue and hard drinking can make the problem even worse.

Severe swelling around the eyes, though, may be due to allergy, Dr. Burkholder says, particularly in young people.

Remedies?

An hour or so in an upright position normally will settle things if a dependent position has been to blame, and cold compresses (ice cubes wrapped in a towel) can speed recovery if you're pressed for time to look your best. (For allergies, it's best to see an allergist or an ophthalmologist.) And for hard drinking and fatigue, a couple of early nights back-to-back would be well worth a try.

Q/ Does alcohol cause cancer?

A/ It can, particularly in heavy smokers, but the risks for people who do not smoke—and who do not overimbibe—appear to be quite small. A researcher from the Department of Epidemiology at the Harvard School of Public Health looked into the issue from a statistical standpoint recently, and this is what he found:

"For the four sites for which there is substantial evidence for a carcinogenic role of alcohol [the mouth, the esophagus, the larynx, and the liver], there was a total of 15,029 cancers in U.S. men in 1974, and 5,318 cancers in women. Of these, I estimate that approximately 8,424 cases in men and about 2,648 cases in women can be attributed to alcohol, for a total of about 11,100 cases."

Computing this figure of 11,100 against the total number of cancers *of all types* recorded in the United States in 1974 (365,532), he determined that the proportion of alcohol-related cases came to a relatively scant 3 percent. He emphasized, too, "that most of the effect of alcohol seems to be concentrated among those who consume alcohol regularly and heavily.

"Antismoking programs would probably be more effective than antidrinking campaigns in preventing cancer attributed to alcohol because of the double jeopardy effect between these two carcinogens," he said.

Q/ How many days of exercise can I miss before I begin to lose the fitness I've gained?

A/ "Once you've achieved a moderate level of fitness, you can afford to miss about three," says exercise physiologist Jack Mahurin, Ph.D., of Springfield College. "After that, muscular strength and cardiopulmonary gains begin to revert. And studies show that we begin to lose from our richest areas first."

If you're a runner, for example, and you've developed great lung power, a loss in wind is what you'll notice before a loss in muscular strength. Or if you've finely tuned a particular set of muscles through weight training, a decrease in performance from them is what will be most noticeable.

"With that 72-hour figure in mind, then, what's an ideal workout schedule for most people?" we asked Dr. Mahurin.

"It's been shown that a well-exhausted muscle needs a minimum of 48 hours to thoroughly rebuild itself," Dr. Mahurin said. "Which is why workouts every other day—if they're strenuous—is what we recommend."

"But then how can world-class marathoners get away with working out *twice* a day, *every* day?" we asked.

"Because they're still obeying a hard/easy-day principle," Dr. Mahurin explained. "They may be working out every day, but they're not pushing themselves every day. They've gotten themselves to a level of fitness where what may seem like a hard workout for most people is actually an easy one for them."

Exertion, in other words, depends on who's doing the exerting.

And how long a layoff could *you* take before you would lose *everything* you had worked for?

Depending on the level of fitness from which your descent began, studies indicate somewhere between five weeks and two months.

Q/ Can sex affect athletic performance?

A/ Yes, but for better as well as for worse. According to Gabe Mirkin, M.D., for players "uptight" the night before a game, former coach of the New York Jets Weeb Ewbank actually used to recommend it. Sleep is what's important before competition, and if sex helps you get it, fine.

"It's not so much sex that hurts some of these guys as it is the staying up all night looking for it," Casey Stengel once said. And in the opinion of the AMA's Committee on the Medical Aspects of Sports, the only other way sex might slow you down would be "if you believed it would."

Physically, in other words, there is no evidence whatsoever that it has to. "To restrict a player from having sex before a game would be hogwash," world-famous sex specialist William Masters, M.D., has said. "An athlete burns up more energy in a pregame warm-up."

Dr. Craig Sharp, Britain's chief medical advisor at the 1972 Olympics, tells of two runners who would seem to have taken Dr. Masters to heart. One, a middle-distance specialist, set a world record within an hour of having had sex. The other, a miler similarly charged, covered his course in a personal best of four minutes flat.

Not all, however, are fortunate enough to be so affected. As one marathon runner has reported to Dr. Mirkin, author of *The Sportsmedicine Book* (Little, Brown, 1978), "When I run after sex my legs are heavy, and having timed myself over a 20-mile course, I'm consistently a full six minutes slower on mornings I've indulged." And in the words of a professional hockey player —one less fortunate than a teammate accustomed to relations prior to face-off—"I tried it and found my legs so rubbery I didn't know what I was doing on the ice. There was no way I could recover—even two hours after making love."

Be your own judge. Rest assured, however, whatever you decide, that it's been the experience of most that sex—particularly if spaced a night in advance—need be no detriment to athletic performance whatsoever.

Q/ Are there any advantages to using margarine instead of butter?

A/ Better words to use than "advantages" here might be "fewer hazards." Because with butter and margarine there *are* no advantages. Only *dis*advantages.

Both are highly concentrated sources of fat—50 percent saturated, 23 percent monosaturated, and 3 percent polyunsaturated in the case of butter;

Nutritive Content
of Butter vs. Margarine

	Butter (100 grams)	Margarine (100 grams)
Water (percent)	15.9	15.7
Calories	717	719
Protein (grams)	0.9	0.9
Fat (grams)	81.1	80.5
Carbohydrates (grams)	0.1	0.9
Cholesterol (milligrams)	219	0
Fiber (grams)	0	(NA)
Ash (milligrams)	2.1	2.0
Calcium (milligrams)	24.0	29.9
Phosphorus (milligrams)	23.0	22.9
Potassium (milligrams)	26.0	42.4
Sodium (milligrams)	826	943
Magnesium (milligrams)	2.0	2.6
Iron (milligrams)	0.2	(NA)
Zinc (milligrams)	0.1	(NA)
Vitamin A (I.U.)	3,058	3,307
Vitamin C (milligrams)	0	0.2
Thiamine (milligrams)	0.005	0.010
Riboflavin (milligrams)	0.034	0.037
Niacin (milligrams)	0.042	0.023
Folate (micrograms)	3.0	1.2

NOTES: NA—information not available.
I.U.—international units.
One stick of butter or margarine weighs about 113 grams.
Unsalted butter contains 11 milligrams of sodium per 100 grams.

SOURCE: Adapted from U.S. Department of Agriculture Handbook no. 8–4.

about 13 percent saturated, 45 percent monosaturated and 18 percent polyunsaturated in the case of corn oil margarine.

We mention these figures because it is believed by most of the scientific community that saturated fats raise cholesterol, that polyunsaturated fats lower it, and that monosaturated fats have no effect either way. Hence, the current recommendations that we switch to the largely polyunsaturated fats in margarine.

Recently, however, there has emerged a small but very outspoken group of researchers who want the blame for heart disease shared by another class of fats—partially hydrogenated fats (which are abundant in margarine).

A similar situation exists in regard to fats and cancer. Most research suggests that fats—of *any* kind—pose a risk. And here again, the researchers who are down on partially hydrogenated fats for causing heart disease are also down on them for promoting cancer. The fats in margarine, they say, are contributing as much—if not *more*—to cancer risk than the others.

From this cloud of controversy, however, emerges at least one inarguable point: Fat is to be avoided—whether it be in the form of butter, margarine, mayonnaise, salad oil, bacon, whipped cream, or whatever.

Q/ What causes shin splints?

A/ Shin splints are pains in the muscles around the area of the shin bones. They can be caused by running or jumping on hard surfaces, or simply by overuse. You know you have them if pain worsens when you go to stand on your toes.

The best way to relieve the discomfort of shin splints is to ice them, elevate them, and rest them. Beyond that, shoes with good heel support and shock absorption, running on softer surfaces, avoiding hills, and trying to run slightly more back on your heels could help.

Exercises can correct the basic muscle imbalance that causes shin splints in the first place. Sit on a table with your legs hanging over the sides and flex your foot to lift a weight (a paint can weighing several pounds will do) that you have draped over your toes. Then stretch your calf muscles by putting your hands straight ahead of you against a wall and slowly moving your feet backwards—as far as you can go—while still keeping your heels on the ground.

Shin splints occur most often in people unaccustomed to training, but they also can plague experienced athletes (such as distance runners) when they switch to lighter shoes, harder surfaces, or concentrated speed work.

Q/ Can sunbathing cause skin cancer?

A/ Yes, especially if you overdo it. A sunburn is, in effect, a radiation burn caused by the middle wavelengths of the sun's ultraviolet rays. They are strongest during the middle part of the day—between 10:00 A.M. and 2:00 P.M.—and most dangerous in areas close to the equator.

Is there a way to tan safely?

Not really. A tanned skin is a damaged skin, most experts agree. The FDA's Bureau of Radiological Health has shown that ultraviolet radiation can affect the ability of your skin's cells to reproduce themselves.

Genetic material known as DNA is what gets burned, and while most of the time cells can bounce back, there are times when they can't. They either die, which makes your skin look old, or they continue on as mutations. And it's these mutations that can lead to cancer. Not right away, scientists say, but later. Skin cancers in people under 20 are rare; it's not until you reach 70 that your "healthy" tan is likely to catch up with you.

So go easy on the browning this summer. And know when you're "under fire" and when you're not.

- Ultraviolet rays *do* pass through water—so you're not as safe swimming as you may think.
- Rays, however, do *not* pass through sand. Roughly one-third of the exposure you get while beaching is by way of reflection.
- Cloud covers, depending on thickness, can provide some protection—but not much. A thin cover might weaken sunlight by 20 percent, meaning you get cooked in 30 minutes instead of 20.
- Lotions can soothe a burn, but not prevent one. You need a *sunscreen* to block ultraviolet rays, the best of which contain a B complex vitamin called para-aminobenzoic acid—or PABA. It lets just enough rays through to let you look rosy—but not roasted.

Have fun in the sun this summer, but be careful. An estimated 80 percent of all skin cancers are sun or sunlamp related. Ultraviolet beauty is *not* a sign of health.

Q/ Is roller-skating good exercise?

A/ Like a lot of other activities, it depends on how you go about it. If you skate hard enough to maintain a heart rate of 70 percent of what you're capable (220 minus your age), and you do it continuously for at least 30 minutes three times a week, then yes, roller-skating is *very* good exercise. We say "very" because it's a lot easier on weight-bearing joints than running, racquetball, and tennis.

Providing, of course, you learn how to fall. The idea is to stay relaxed and avoid landing on sparsely padded spots like elbows and coccyx. Knee, elbow, and maybe even seat cushions are a good idea—even once you think you're pretty good.

Choosing the right skates is also important, says Allen Selner, M.D., a podiatrist from Los Angeles. He advises buying a brand that offers half sizes to ensure a precise fit, and choosing leather rather than vinyl uppers to allow feet to breathe. Absorbent cotton socks are his recommendation for handling the problem of sweating.

Figure on burning about 660 calories per hour when you wheel with gusto. You employ basically the same leg muscles when you skate as you do skiing (the quadriceps, or front thigh muscles), so if you're looking for a way to get ready for the slopes, roller-skating could be it—falls and all.

Q/ Does air conditioning filter out pollution?

A/ No, and if your unit is old, it may even be *adding* pollutants. Room air conditioners contain filters capable of pulling out particles of dust, but as for the more minute villains contributed by industrial wastes and automobile exhaust, these more serious pollutants are being cooled (and dehumidified) at best.

The problem with air conditioning units is that despite being made of aluminum, they can corrode—and this corrosion tends to get circulated into the air in the form of a very minute dust—a nuisance to your lungs and your janitor, both.

Air conditioners can be of some value in removing pollen from the air for hay fever sufferers—but even here, the effects are minimal.

What you need to really clean the air is an air filtration system. They come in various sizes for use in factories, offices, and homes, and are available from a number of manufacturers. Units vary according to efficiency—the best remove particles as tiny as 0.01 micron. Be sure to check closely on the capabilities of a unit before buying.

Q/ Do light beers contain less alcohol than regular beers?

A/ Generally speaking, yes. Just how much less, though, depends on the beer.
Gablinger's, for example, purports to be nearly as potent as most nor-

mally brewed beers at 3.2 percent alcohol by weight. Schlitz Light, by contrast, tips the scales at a relatively demure 2.96 percent (see table). And yet both contain the same number of calories—about 96 per 12 ounces.

How can that be?

Each brewery has its own recipe for "lightening." Some selectively change the proportion of raw materials (malt, hops, yeast, and carbohydrate sources called adjuncts) per volume of water right from the start, while others concentrate more on removing residual carbohydrates (in the form of nonfermentable grain sugars) after fermentation has taken place. It is this latter method that tends to leave alcohol contents more in line with normally brewed beers.

Alcohol and Calories in Beer

	Percent Alcohol by Weight	Calories*
Michelob Regular	4.00	163
Budweiser	3.72	150
Miller High Life	3.2–4.0	150
Schlitz	3.78	146
Coors Regular	3.54	142
Michelob Light	3.25	134
Natural Light	3.28	110
Coors Light	3.32	102
Gablinger's	3.2	96
Miller Lite	3.2–4.0	96
Schlitz Light	2.96	9.
Schmidt's Light	3.2	9

NOTE: *Per 12 ounces of beer cited.

SOURCE: Information supplied by companies.

Q/ When's the best time to take vitamins?

A/ The fat-soluble vitamins (A, D, and E) should be taken with your largest meal of the day, "because that's usually when the greatest amount of fat is present in the stomach to aid their absorption," according to Stephen Paul, Ph.D., of Temple University's School of Pharmacy.

As for the water-soluble vitamins (C and the B's), "these, too, should be taken with food, either during a meal itself or within a half hour before or after," Dr. Paul said. "Vitamins act as catalysts to help you use food more efficiently. So it's best to get the two together."

For this reason, Dr. Paul recommends never taking vitamins in place of food. That goes for minerals, too.

A word on vitamin C. Because there's a limit to how much your body can absorb, you're better off taking C periodically during the day, instead of a single dose.

Q/ Why don't women body builders develop muscles as big as men's?

A/ The answer to that lies in the hormone testosterone, which "is found in much higher levels in normal men than in normal women," says Edward L. Fox, Ph.D., director of the Laboratory of Work Physiology at Ohio State University and author of *Sports Physiology* (W. B. Saunders, 1979). That is *not* to say, however, that women do not get stronger, fitter, and firmer by training with weights. They simply enjoy these benefits *without* experiencing the increase in muscle *size* that men do, as the graph shows.

As you can see, increases in muscle girth (circumference) were in every case greater in the men than in the women, with the largest increase registered by women being 0.6 centimeter, or just less than a quarter of an inch.

"Such small increases," says Dr. Fox, "clearly demonstrate that muscular hypertrophy [growth] in the female as a result of weight training programs will certainly not lead to excessive muscular bulk or produce a masculinizing effect." Women do, nonetheless, "respond to weight resistance programs with increases in strength and muscular endurance."

Comparative Weight Training Results in Men and Women

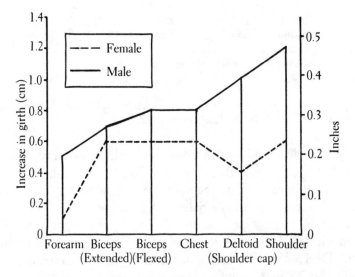

Results of a weight training program in which women made the same relative gains in strength as men, but without similar gains in muscular size.

SOURCE: Reprinted from *Sports Physiology*, by Edward L. Fox (Philadelphia: W. B. Saunders, 1979). Used with permission of W. B. Saunders.

Q/ What's the difference between high-density lipoproteins (HDLs) and low-density lipoproteins (LDLs)?

A/ Both are microscopic particles in your bloodstream that carry cholesterol, but whereas HDLs carry cholesterol off to the liver for disposal, LDLs pass it around to cells and dump it off to clog the arteries. It is better, obviously, to have more high-density lipoproteins than low ones.

HDL and LDL levels, to a degree, are inherited. But recent studies show that by exercising regularly, not smoking, and, perhaps, by drinking only in moderation, HDL levels *can* be increased.

As for the effects of diet on HDL, the recommendation here seems to be: Put less of a strain on the HDLs you *do* have by avoiding fatty foods in the first place.

Low HDL levels are considered a major risk factor in heart disease. So if you're not very active, or you smoke, or you eat a lot of fatty foods, have your levels checked. If the amount of total cholesterol in your blood is between seven and nine times the amount of cholesterol being carried by HDLs, your risk of suffering a heart attack is twice as great as someone whose ratio of total cholesterol to HDLs is average (5 for men, 4.5 for women). A ratio of 13 or more *triples* your chances.

Q/ Am I wasting my time exercising just once a week?

A/ No, not entirely. Michael L. Pollock, Ph.D., professor of medicine at the University of Wisconsin School of Medicine–Mount Sinai Medical Center in Milwaukee, did a study several years ago which showed that aerobic capacity improved by 8 percent in men who exercised just once a week. Dr. Pollock had them jogging at heart rates of 85 to 95 percent of their maximum capacities for periods of 30 minutes. He also measured the improved aerobic capacity of men who went through this same workout three and five times a week. Their improvements measured 13 percent and 17 percent, respectively. So in terms of aerobic capacity improvement, you get what you pay for.

With weight loss, however, Dr. Pollock found a slightly different story. Exercising just once a week had no effect whatsoever on body weight or fat. Exercising *twice* a week didn't either, even when men logged as much as four miles per workout. Only when exercise sessions came at least *three times* a week did any of Dr. Pollock's subjects begin to lose weight. "It appears that a minimum of three days per week is necessary to develop cardiovascular-respiratory fitness *and* to show significant changes in body weight and fat," he concluded. Hence the three-day minimum prescribed by most fitness experts.

How about more than three days?

Up to five days, Dr. Pollock has found, will continue to bestow proportionate benefits. But with five, for some people, come problems. "In one study we conducted on young adult men training one, three, or five days per week, we found that the rate of injury for the five-day-per-week group was *three times* that of the three-day-per-week group," Dr. Pollock said. "It appears that the body needs sufficient rest between workouts, and that a day off between days of jogging may protect a participant—especially a beginner—from injury. If one wants to exercise more frequently," Dr. Pollock advises, "jogging should be interspersed with days of walking, bicycling, swimming, or some other activity that does not cause continual pounding on the legs."

Q/ Is it harder on my liver to drink moderately every day—or heavily, but only on weekends?

A/ "The person who drinks continuously is at a greater risk of liver damage than the binge drinker who stops to allow his liver a chance to recover," says Martin Swerdlow, M.D., chairman of the Department of Pathology at Michael Reese Hospital and Medical Center in Chicago.

A look at how the liver is affected by alcohol illustrates why that is true. The liver performs a variety of important digestive functions, not the least of which is breaking down the fats we eat. But when we throw alcohol into the picture, this function gets put on hold. First order of business becomes detoxifying this alcoholic onslaught by turning it into carbon dioxide and water, a process which takes all the energy the liver can muster. As a result, fat metabolism lags, and fatty deposits, as they wait their turn, begin to collect on the liver's beleaguered exterior.

If this sort of logjam happens only occasionally, there is no great problem. The liver simply lets some of the fat enter the bloodstream, and the rest it gets around to metabolizing eventually. Create this overload too often, however, and you wind up coating your liver with a layer of fat thick enough to impair its function.

When asked how *much* one would have to drink daily to bring this situation about, Dr. Swerdlow could not be specific. "Susceptibility for liver disease depends on the person," he said. The capacity for metabolizing alcohol, the ability of liver cells to regenerate themselves, body weight, and eating habits—all are contributing factors. But anything over the equivalent of 80 grams of alcohol a day (day after day for many years), he said, would "definitely" increase one's chances. (That's about five shots of 80-proof whiskey, 70 ounces of beer, or 30 ounces of wine.)

A somewhat less permissive quota comes from Charles S. Lieber, M.D., professor of medicine and pathology at the Mount Sinai School of Medicine in New York. He says liver damage can occur after only two days of drinking between 7 and 13 shots of hard liquor. Put that in the perspective of a lifetime and you begin to see why drinking daily extends liver disease such a cordial welcome.

Is there such a thing as a "safe" daily limit? "We think that maybe 0.7 gram for every kilogram of body weight may be a safe level," says Thomas Turner, M.D., dean emeritus of the medical faculty at the Johns Hopkins University School of Medicine. That figures out to be—based on a weight of 176 pounds—6 ounces of 80-proof liquor, 20 ounces of wine (12 percent alcohol), or 53 ounces of beer (4½ percent alcohol).

Q/ Does it help, when trying to lose weight, to wear a sweat suit or to exercise when it's hot?

A/ No, and it can be dangerous. You'll sweat more, of course. But sweat is not melted fat. It's water, with a little sodium and some potassium thrown in. And you only drink it right back.

The secret of losing weight is to *burn* calories, not dissolve them. And it's work, not discomfort, that does it. You may *feel* like you've done more work inside a sweat suit, but chances are you've *done* less. Muscles just don't perform as well "boiled over." Like your car engine, they have an optimum temperature at which they prefer to perform, and it's considerably less than the inferno that a rubber sweat suit on a hot day can produce.

Sweat comes to the surface of your skin for a reason: to be evaporated and cool you. Suffocate yourself in sweat gear and you choke off the air flow needed to do that. Excessive humidity can do the same thing.

Better to run four miles comfortably in shorts than to hobble through three in sweats, for the "fatigue" produced by overheating is not a true reflection of the amount of energy you've actually put out. And the dangers of heat stroke are very real. If you begin to feel light-headed or you stop perspiring, head for home, slowly.

Play it cool during the summer. Exercise hard if you want, but do it in the morning or early evening, and in a minimum of clothing. Dress like a mummy and you may wind up one. And try to fit more potassium into your diet. On a hot day you can lose your daily supply of this important mineral through sweating alone. Fresh fruits and vegetables are the best sources of replacement potassium because they're low in sodium and fat. The much publicized sports tonics are also good, as are fruit and tomato juice, and beer! Don't worry about salt. You don't lose that much when you sweat, and there's plenty in the food you eat.

Keep cool, drink right, eat light, and exercise.

Q/ How much protein does the body really need?

A/ Less than most Americans get. One four-ounce serving of a high-quality protein (such as meat) in conjunction with a well-balanced diet of fruits, vegetables, dairy products, and grains is all the average adult really needs. But he gets more, and the excess usually does more harm than good by getting stored as fat.

Joan Ullyot, M.D., author of *Running Free* (G. P. Putnam's Sons, 1980) has found that the healthiest blood chemistries are those common to runners who are vegetarians. This group, she says, is followed by sedentary vegetarians, followed by meat-eating runners. The blood of the average, inactive, meat-loving American, she says, is in pretty bad shape. High in fat of the worst kind.

Protein may be said to come in two forms—high quality, and low. Animal proteins (including meat, poultry, dairy products, and eggs) are all high, meaning they contain all eight of the amino acids essential to the building and repair of body tissue. But they also contain saturated fat—the kind that is solid at room temperature and bad for the heart.

Vegetarians make do on low-quality proteins—the kind found in plants. Low-quality proteins are deficient in one or more of the essential amino acids, so they have to be eaten in the right combinations. Rice and beans, for example. Individually, each is lacking. But together, they're dynamite—as potent as porterhouse, and high in fiber, carbohydrates, and a lot of vitamins and minerals not found in meat. Well-planned vegetarianism can make for exceptionally healthful fare.

If you're leaning that way, or are concerned about the amount of animal fat in your diet, take a look at Frances Moore Lappe's *Diet for a Small Planet* (Ballantine, 1975). It's probably the best book on the subject to date, simply written but informative. You'll be amazed at how much protein there is around, once you've learned where to look for it.

Q/ Some of my friends are urging me to try cocaine. Is it dangerous?

A/ The answer to that question depends on whom you ask. According to the National Commission on Reform of the Federal Criminal Laws:

"Cocaine is a powerful stimulant. While it does not cause physical dependence, a very strong psychological dependence upon cocaine can be developed. It should be classified as a dangerous drug because it may precipitate acute anxiety and psychotic episodes, and there is a strong possibility that such episodes may involve aggression or violent behavior."

Noted professor and author Andrew Weil, M.D., however, disagrees.

"Among the hundreds of cocaine users I have known, I have seen the drug induce only good moods. It would appear that many of the beliefs about cocaine that have led to current law-enforcement practices are unfounded and have their origin in the hysterical fears of past days when cocaine was judged guilty by association, particularly with opiate addicts."

Dr. Weil goes on to explain, however, "in defending cocaine against the attacks of misinformed persons, I do not mean to suggest that the drug is innocuous or in any way beneficial. I see two main problems with it.

"The first is simply that cocaine does not miraculously bestow energy on the body. It merely releases energy that is already stored chemically in certain parts of the nervous system. Consequently, when the immediate effect of the drug wears off, one feels 'down'—less energetic than normal."

The second problem, Dr. Weil says, is that "tolerance to the high of cocaine develops rapidly, so that a second dose gives a less intense effect that lasts a shorter time. Users who have access to large amounts of cocaine can find themselves, very quickly, using it all the time . . ."

And that can become a problem, Dr. Weil says, because "over a long time, snorting cocaine . . . leads to local weakening of [nasal] tissue by interference with blood supply. Rare individuals who use it in great excess may even develop perforations of the nasal septum [the plate of bone and cartilage that divides the inside of the nose]."

As a "final and troublesome problem" with cocaine, Dr. Weil cites "the difficulty of leaving it alone. It is terribly hard for people who like the stimulation of cocaine to let the drug sit around unused. The white powder seems to exert a strong attraction even if it is kept out of sight" (*The Marriage of the Sun and the Moon*, Houghton Mifflin, 1980).

Q/ Why am I going bald, and what can I do about it?

A/ You're going bald because one of your ancestors did, and short of a hair transplant there really isn't much you can do about it. You can improve the quality of the hair you do have, through good nutrition and proper care, but you can't, unfortunately, fight genetics.

The total number of hair follicles in an adult has been estimated at five million, 150,000 of which are in the scalp. As dividing cells at the bottom of the hair follicle are pushed upward, they eventually die and become the visible product we know as hair. Hair, then, is actually dead tissue composed of protein, and it's the follicle, lying beneath the scalp, that's alive and nurturing the growing.

In humans, each follicle grows hair in cycles, the duration of which depends on where that follicle is located on the body. On the scalp, for example, a hair normally grows steadily for two to six years, at which point it stops, and after three to four months is shed. Following a "rest" period, the process begins all over again, except if that follicle has gotten the notion to call it quits, in which case you're left with a spot we call . . . "bald."

Scalp hair grows at the rate of about one-third of a millimeter a day—one inch every two to three months—which, with 150,000 hairs to consider, amounts to roughly 175 feet of solid protein a day—12 miles a year.

So-called "male pattern" thinning, seen earliest at the temples and over the top of the scalp, is very common in men, but similar thinning may occur in women.

Normally we lose between 20 and 60 scalp hairs a day as old hairs are shed to make room for the new, but this rate can be affected by various events. Childbirth, for example, or a major illness, or even surgical procedure. Blood loss, severe emotional stress, even rapid weight loss diets or protein deficiencies can cause hair to come out literally by the handful—though under most circumstances the loss is only temporary, with growth returning to normal once all is well.

Hair transplants involve relocating skin in which hair is healthy to areas where others have quit. The most common approach uses four-millimeter "plugs" of hair-bearing skin. Most do fairly well, normally producing 12 to 18 healthy hairs each.

As for hair care, rinses containing protein can fill in defects on the surface of hair shafts, making them smoother and thicker, but they do nothing for the health of your hair internally, and the effects are temporary at best.

Q/ What causes blisters and how should they be treated?

A/ A blister is caused when rubbing of skin against skin (or skin against equipment) causes the layers of the epidermis to separate and fill with a clear fluid provided by blood vessels deeper down. A blood blister is formed when further wear breaks down into these blood vessels themselves. Older people are more likely to develop blisters than young, and men (for reasons unknown) are more prone to develop them than women.

Heat and dampness accelerate the blistering process. Blisters form most easily where skin is held firmly in place by underlying connective tissue (palms, soles, and nipples), and in the parts of your body where the blood pressure is greatest—like the feet.

Blisters on the underside of the foot are usually due to side-to-side movement caused by wearing shoes that are too wide; blisters that develop on the tops of the toes, on the other hand, are normally the result of shoes being too narrow.

As for blisters of the heels, they tend to develop on the sides of heels if heels are narrow. A stick-on felt substance called moleskin (available at most drugstores) is a good way to shore up the heel area of shoes that are "wobbly."

The best way to treat a blister is to drain it. Drainage permits the separated skin layers of most blisters (about 90 percent) to grow back together—usually within about four days, whereas only about 20 percent ever heal themselves in this way if left "bubbled."

Draining should be done very carefully by inserting a sterile needle into the edge of the bubbled area and pressing gently to force out the fluid. The entire area should first be cleaned with alcohol, and immediately after surgery the damaged skin should be covered with tape.

If the sore refills itself, poke it again. You may have to do this three or four times within a period of 24 hours.

If the blister has broken—and drained itself—sterilize the area with an antibiotic ointment before applying tape. The ointment will fight infection and also tend to keep the tape from sticking.

The U.S. Army says that blisters cause one out of every ten recruits to miss at least three days of basic training. They're a very common problem —but not inescapable. The secret is to avoid circumstances conducive to their development in the first place.

Q/ If carrying extra fat around is a burden on the heart, why isn't carrying extra muscle stressful also?

A/ That's a good question, with several good answers.

First, muscle (unlike fat) earns its keep. The amount of exercise you have to do—not only to build muscle, but also to *keep* it—is enough to keep your heart in shape to deal with it. Fat, by comparison, is often the result of a *lack* of physical activity. And hence the heart that has to carry a lot of fat is apt to be insufficiently trained for the task.

Second, whereas muscle facilitates movement, fat impedes it. To use an automotive analogy, adding extra fat to your body is like putting sandbags in your trunk, while adding muscle is like investing in the additional weight of a more efficient transmission. The added weight of muscle is more than offset by the degree to which it makes it easier for your body—and hence your heart—to go about its daily business. Add enough *fat* to your body, on the other hand, and you wind up making bodily movement difficult.

Then, too, muscle contains more blood vessels than fat, making it easier for blood to circulate. An analogy here might be a sprinkler nozzle you put on the end of a garden hose: One with five holes would make for a greater buildup of pressure than one with 25. And so it is with blood trying to make its way through your body. It meets with more resistance as it makes its way through fat than it does through muscle, and this resistance gets distributed throughout the entire circulatory system. Which is why obesity and high blood pressure go hand in hand. Excess fat creates resistance that need not —and should not—be.

Q/ Is it possible to "spot reduce"?

A/ No. Just as it is impossible to control where fat will go when you put it *on*, it's impossible to dictate where it will come *off* when you lose it. Fat loss depends on the total number of calories you expend, *not* where you expend them. And if there is any predictable pattern at all to weight loss, it is that fat seems to come off those areas *first* where it has been gained *last*. With these unfortunate truths in mind, let's look at the inefficiency of doing sit-ups, for example, to take fat off the waist.

A full half hour of sit-ups, depending on how big you are and how fast you do them, might burn 120 to 150 calories. Jogging, cycling, or swimming, by comparison, might burn *two times* that many, and hence be *twice* as good a way to lose fat from the belly, as a result. The larger the muscle exercised, the more calories burned. And so the best muscles of all for "spot reducing," wherever those spots may be, are the legs.

That is not to say that localized exercises of lesser muscle groups go wasted. They *do* burn calories, and they also can provide greater muscle tone to areas which may appear fatter than they actually are simply because of sagging.

When it comes to losing actual fat, though, there is no better way than to burn it off. And the muscles that burn best are the big ones.

Q/ How long does it take to get fit?

A/ Probably not as long as you think. If you're healthy and are willing to invest about 20 minutes a day, you should be able to reach an initial level of fitness in only about two weeks. We base that answer on an experiment done recently by a doctor in Australia.

John Pearn, M.D., put 50 untrained male college students through 20 minutes of exercise a day—and in only *14 days* "all the subjects became fit . . . with objective improvement in both absolute strength and pulse recovery times." The men's muscle strength increased by 29 to 30 percent, and their endurance (cardiovascular power) increased by 15 to 25 percent. Dr. Pearn's program consisted of three sets of ten exercises (among them the Harvard step test, chin-ups, and weight lifting) which the men went through as quickly as they comfortably could (in most cases about ten minutes) twice a day. Total exercise time over the two-week period came to only about six hours (*British Medical Journal,* December 6, 1980).

"The interpretation of this finding," Dr. Pearn concluded, "is that six hours of circuit training [going quickly from one exercise to another] spread evenly over 14 days will achieve a mean increase in physical fitness . . . irrespective of initial enthusiasm and motivation." (To test the importance of the motivation factor in becoming fit, Dr. Pearn had included in his study 30 students who were not initially interested in getting into shape. And yet these students achieved the same results as the students who were motivated.)

Dr. Pearn's experiment should come as good news to anyone having trouble getting started on a fitness program.

Q/ Is salt bad for people who don't have high blood pressure?

A/ Possibly not. For people *not* genetically susceptible to developing high blood pressure by middle age (roughly 80 to 90 percent of the population), average daily sodium intake (estimated to be between 3,900 and 4,700 milligrams) does not appear to be dangerous. But . . .

There is no clearcut way of knowing in advance whether or not you are among this genetically protected majority. Which is why an easy hand on the saltshaker—for everybody—is a good idea.

Two hundred milligrams of sodium (the amount in one-tenth teaspoon of salt) is all the body really needs. This amount is helpful in maintaining the pressure and volume of the blood within normal ranges, and also in assisting the transmission of nerve impulses. Anything substantially beyond this amount—in normal people—gets excreted via the bowels, urinary tract, and sweat glands.

In an estimated 10 to 20 percent of people with high blood pressure, however, this excess sodium (for reasons not yet fully understood) gets retained in the blood where it encourages water retention, and hence high blood pressure. High blood pressure, also known as hypertension, is a known risk factor in heart disease and stroke.

An encouraging note for this 10 to 20 percent of hypertensives, however, is that high blood pressure can be prevented—*and even corrected*—if sodium intakes are kept low: below about 1,400 milligrams a day. (That is the amount in about three-quarters teaspoon of salt.)

In light of these findings, you're best off—even if your blood pressure is normal—to avoid salt when you can. There is more sodium than you need in the food you eat (see the following table). And considering how salt makes you thirsty (which can lead to consuming excess calories in the form of

Sodium Content of Selected Foods

	Portion	Sodium (milligrams)
Ham	3 ounces	1,114
Dill pickle	1	928
American cheese	2 ounces	812
Blue cheese	2 ounces	792
Canadian bacon	1 slice	394
Soy sauce	1 teaspoon	343
Green olives	4	323
Bacon, cooked	2 slices	274
Peanuts, dry-roasted, salted	¼ cup	247
Salt	⅛ teaspoon	242
Milk	1 cup	122
Butter	1 tablespoon	116
Ice cream, vanilla	1 cup	112
Cod, broiled with butter	3 ounces	93
Cream cheese	2 tablespoons	82
Egg, raw	1	59
Beet greens, cooked	½ cup	55
Spinach, cooked	½ cup	47
Beets, cooked	½ cup	37
Artichoke	1 medium	36
Carrot, raw	1 medium	34
Celery, raw	1 stalk	25
Kale, cooked	½ cup	24
Broccoli, raw	1 medium stalk	23
Sweet potato, baked	1 medium	20
Honeydew melon	⅛	18
Mustard greens, cooked	½ cup	13
Cantaloupe	¼ medium	12
Collard greens, cooked	½ cup	12
Parsnips, cooked	½ cup	10
Green pepper, raw or cooked	1 medium	9
Cabbage, cooked	½ cup	8
Cauliflower, cooked	½ cup	7
Brussels sprouts, raw	4	4
Radishes	3	2

SOURCE: Adapted from *The Sodium Content of Your Food*, Home and Garden Bulletin no. 233 (Washington, D.C.: Science and Education Administration, U.S. Department of Agriculture, 1980).

liquids) and arouses the appetite (another encouragement for overconsumption), you're best off to leave salt in its shaker.

Q/ Are there vitamins I can take for healthier hair?

A/ There is evidence that the B vitamins, vitamin E, and the mineral zinc all can contribute to healthy hair, but perhaps most effective of all in promoting shinier, thicker locks is gelatin. One experiment involving 52 people showed that supplementing their diet with 14 grams (about seven teaspoons) of unflavored gelatin a day increased the diameter of individual hair strands by as much as 45 percent in two months (*Nutrition Reports International,* June, 1976).

But is thick hair healthy hair?

Yes, the experts say. The gelatin-induced increase constituted "an improvement in the mechanical properties of the hair," the researchers said. When the volunteers stopped eating their gelatin, however, their hair reverted to its original girth within six months.

With that in mind, we offer the following hair "tonic" that you might think about ingesting on a daily basis. It contains protein, choline, inositol, pantothenate, biotin, vitamin E, and zinc—virtually everything a head of hair could ask for. Whipped up in a blender, the cocktail can serve as a nutritious breakfast or a hearty nightcap. If its taste doesn't thrill you, play around with it a bit using fruited yogurt, perhaps, instead of plain, and maybe a little less brewer's yeast (which is not, admittedly, known for its gourmet appeal).

1	cup plain yogurt
1	banana
½	cup berries
3	tablespoons wheat germ
2	tablespoons brewer's yeast
1	tablespoon lecithin granules
1	teaspoon vitamin C crystals
1	raw egg yolk
1	envelope (1 tablespoon) unflavored gelatin powder
	honey to taste (optional)

Combine all ingredients and blend until smooth.

Q/ Can too much exercise diminish a man's sex drive?

A/ Not for chemical reasons. It's been found that vigorous exercise actually stimulates the production of the hormone that scientists feel is responsible for the male sex drive in the first place—testosterone.

Dr. J. R. Suttor of the Garvan Institute of Medical Research in Australia measured testosterone levels in two groups of men (athletes and non-athletes) before, during, and after a period of vigorous exercise. He found that the levels of this hormone were greatest *after* the workouts.

These findings can be explained by the fact that testosterone is important in muscular activity. The hormone makes it easier for muscles to store glycogen (their favorite fuel), and so the more active your muscles are, the more testosterone you are apt to have at your disposal—for exercise *or* sex.

Then, too, there's the matter of improved circulation. In someone who is in poor physical condition, the production of testosterone (by the testes) can get discouraged when insufficient blood flow around the gonads fails to distribute the hormone at a healthy rate. (That creates a kind of testosterone logjam to which the testes respond by cutting back on the amount they produce.)

Exercise, if anything, is an aphrodisiac—as many runners happily attest. Its potential for being an obstacle to sex would seem to be restricted to the realm of psychology—those rare cases in which an athlete's training becomes, for whatever reason, virtually all he can think about.

Q/ What effects do steam baths and saunas have on the body?

A/ Exposure to heat in the form of either a steam bath or sauna amounts essentially to a workout for your body's thermal regulation system. Writing in the *Journal of the American Medical Association,* (January 25, 1980), David I. Abramson, M.D., reports that "in normal subjects, there are increases in cardiac output, pulse rate, and central venous pressure, and decreases in circulation time, systolic pressure, and peripheral resistance." What that means is your heart pumps more blood to your skin, for cooling purposes, and less to your internal organs. "There is also a considerable depletion of salt from the body through perspiration," Dr. Abramson notes, "and in hypertensive patients, a noteworthy fall in both systolic and diastolic blood pressures occurs."

As for weight loss, most is dehydration, but the act of sweating in itself *does* burn calories—about 0.6 per gram of water lost, calculates Ward Dean, M.D. That's enough to cost you about 272 calories per pound of water lost.

Relaxation? According to a study done in Finland, you *shouldn't* feel relaxed after a thorough baking because the process elevates concentrations of catecholamines (nervous system stimulants) in the blood. The final effect of this increase, though, may be the stimulation of the well-being center in the brain, the Finnish researchers theorize.

Dr. Abramson views this feeling of relief that follows a steam bath this way: "Perhaps the sense of well-being that occurs after a person leaves the hot, humid environment could be compared with the great feeling of relief experienced by the patient who has been suffering from severe pains and suddenly finds that he has become free of symptoms."

Dr. Abramson feels that steam baths, saunas, and hot tubs should be used by the sound of heart only. "In the presence of any serious organic disability, such as generalized arteriosclerosis, chronic pulmonary disorders, cardiac difficulties, and hyperthyroidism, the sauna and the steam bath are definitely contraindicated," he says. There is also evidence that prolonged saunas, steam baths, and hot tubs should be avoided by women during pregnancy.

As for a steam bath's ability to leach the body of toxins, Dr. Abramson says that's a job better left to the kidneys than the sweat glands.

Q/ Is it dangerous to exercise after a few drinks?

A/ No, but it can be demoralizing. Alcohol is a strange fuel; it supplies energy —but in such a concentrated form that in order to be burned it demands more oxygen than a person exercising is in a position to spare.

It was found, for example, that rats put on a diet containing alcohol needed more oxygen than rats fed a diet that was alcohol-free.

Most adults can safely metabolize about an ounce of 80-proof spirits an hour. At *that* rate, alcohol is a fuel similar—and perhaps even superior (some say)—to food. George Sheehan, M.D., for example, claims that beer consumed in doses of as much as two 12-ounce cans an hour can act as a stimulant and "potent source of calories" for someone running a marathon.

But then beer has some legitimate food value in the form of carbohydrates to pad its blow. Try exercising after a couple of highballs and you ask your system to deal with the effects of alcohol "straight-up." Concentration —as well as rate of consumption—*does* make a difference.

So as you picnic this year, go easy on the refreshments if you want to be a softball hero. You're liable to blow it by coming to the bases loaded.

Q/ How can I avoid a "stitch" when I run?

A/ Side stitch is thought to be caused by the downward tug that running puts on internal organs, and is more apt to occur in someone in less than tip-top shape. Pain usually occurs under the rib cage on the right side, which may be due to the location there of the liver, a solid organ which weighs about four pounds and normally contains one-quarter of the body's total supply of blood.

Stitch can be avoided by:

- *starting out easy.* Breathing heavily—particularly in the beginning of a run—causes stomach muscles to relax, which allows organs inside greater freedom to move about.
- *not running on a full stomach.* By waiting at least an hour and a half for your gut to empty itself, you reduce the weight of the organs being jostled—and hence the strain on the internal devices designed to keep them in place. You also allow your stomach the blood it needs for digestion. (By running while your stomach is digesting, you send some of the blood it needs to the muscles of the legs—and that can cause cramping.)
- *running with a smooth gait.* It's the up and down, bunny rabbit style that's the worst. Try to run as though you're being towed by an invisible rope, keeping head and shoulder movements to a minimum.
- *losing weight.* If you show obvious signs of being plump around the hips and midriff, chances are some of this excess has attached itself to your organs inside—which losing weight will help lighten.
- *doing exercises to strengthen your stomach muscles.* Try bent leg sit-ups or leg lifts. Tightening your stomach muscles will give your innards less room to move around.
- *training consistently.* Very few marathoners have this problem.
- *stretching.* Tight muscles put more of a pull on internal organs.

To relieve a stitch, lie down and breathe deeply. Or if you prefer to remain standing, take deep breaths while bending forward.

Stitch is a very common problem with runners just starting out—so hang in there.

Q/ What is cellulite?

A/ Cellulite is fat upon fat. When fatty tissue builds up to the point where it has to ride piggyback on itself, you wind up with mounds rather than nice smooth marbling.

Why is it crinkly? The dermatologist we talked to explained that when fat builds up to a point where it can't get enough blood, fibrous bands develop that tend to pucker up the softer, healthier portions of flesh like a balloon against a tennis racket.

The best way to get rid of cellulite is the best way to get rid of any fat: Eat less and exercise. You simply have to lose what you can't pump enough blood to keep healthy. Aerobic exercises (such as walking, running, cycling, and swimming) are best because they consume a lot of calories and also improve circulation.

Don't make the mistake of further reducing blood flow to problem areas by squeezing them into armorlike underwear. Cellulite needs all the breathing room it can get, so avoid long periods of sitting, too. If you work at a desk all day, get up every hour or so and move around.

Women, incidentally, are more apt to deposit fat in these kinds of layers than men. It has to do with certain hormonal predispositions—and heredity.

Q/ Is exercise good for bones?

A/ Yes. Bone is living tissue that responds to environmental conditions. When exposed regularly to the strains of exercise, bone (like muscle) adapts by getting thicker, denser, and stronger.

The mechanism responsible for this is called mineralization. As bones are stressed by the muscular contractions and compressional impacts imposed by exercise, they respond by taking on more calcium and phosphorus.

That has been demonstrated in laboratory experiments involving many different types of athletes. Tennis players, for example, were found in one study to have significantly larger wrist and forearm bones in their dominant arms. And middle-aged long-distance runners in another survey proved to have significantly denser leg bones than a group of sedentaries their same age.

In the words of two doctors reporting in *Nutrition Reports International* (June, 1978), "Bone growth and density increase in proportion to the compressional load a bone is asked to carry." Weight lifters, as a result, have been found to have thicker bones than runners, and runners to have thicker bones than swimmers. "A physically active lifestyle above a sedentary level," these authors conclude, "is necessary to induce calcification and stave off the threat of osteoporosis (bone degeneration) in later years."

A study of bedridden hospital patients showed that bones can begin to demineralize when deprived of exercise entirely. Even the moderate strain imposed by the simple act of standing was found in one experiment to retard the rate at which bedridden patients lost bone density. It is important, researchers agree, that people continue to get moderate exercise (such as walking) to maintain skeletal strength as they get older.

Q/ Can I get the fiber I need by eating a high-fiber breakfast cereal?

A/ Yes. Providing the rest of your diet contains at least several servings a day of fruits and/or vegetables, the amount of dietary fiber contained in one serving of most high-fiber cereals can keep your fiber intake at a healthy level.

Kellogg's All-Bran and Bran Buds, Nabisco's 100 Percent Bran and Ralston-Purina's Bran Chex are the highest in fiber. (A mere three able spoons of these supplies the equivalent of about two tablespoons of pure wheat bran—the amount normally recommended by doctors who prescribe bran for laxative purposes.)

Some other brands slightly lower in fiber—but still good sources—are Kellogg's 40 Percent Bran, Raisin Bran, Most, Cracklin' Bran, and Nabisco's Shredded Wheat. The table below should put things in perspective.

Fiber Content of Selected Breakfast Cereals

	Dietary Fiber* (grams)
Unprocessed millers bran	25.6
Nabisco's 100 Percent Bran	22.5
Kellogg's Bran Buds	18.9
Kellogg's All-Bran	16.8
Ralston-Purina Bran Chex	10.0
Kellogg's Cracklin' Bran	9.2
Kellogg's Most	7.6
Kellogg's Toasted Mini-Wheats	6.9
Kellogg's Raisin Bran	6.8
Quaker Oats Corn Bran	6.7
Nabisco's Shredded Wheat	5.3
Kellogg's 40 Percent Bran	5.2
Ralston-Purina Honey Bran	3.9
Quaker Oats Puffed Wheat	1.8

NOTES: *Per cup of cereal cited.
About sugar—To make their regulatory powers palatable, most high-fiber c reals are also high in sugar. With the exceptions of unprocessed millers bran (available in health food stores), Puffed Wheat, Shredded Wheat, and Toasted Mini-Wheats, most are about 20 percent sugar by weight, with Kellogg's Bran Buds leading the pack at 32 percent.

SOURCES: Information supplied by companies. Values also adapted from *McCance and Widdowson's The Composition of Foods*, by A. A. Paul and D. A. T. Southgate (New York: Elsevier/North-Holland Biomedical Press, 1978).

Q/ Is weight training a good way to lose weight?

A/ That depends on what you mean by losing weight if you're talking about weighing less on your bathroom scale, then no, weight training is not a good way to reduce. But if you're interested in turning fat to muscle, it's excellent.

Larry R. Gettman, Ph.D., and Michael L. Pollock, Ph.D., recently reviewed 11 major weight-lifting studies done during the past eight years. They found that, in each one, participants increased their muscle mass (by an average of 2.2 to 7 pounds), decreased their amount of body fat (by between 0.8 and 2.9 percent), improved their strength (by 7 to 32 percent), and improved their cardiovascular (heart and lung) capacities by an average of 5 percent (*Physician and Sportsmedicine*, January, 1981).

That last figure did not compare all that favorably with more aerobic programs of similar intensity and duration (such as running/jogging, walking/hiking, swimming, skating, cycling, rope-skipping, and cross-country skiing —which have been shown to increase cardiovascular fitness by 15 to 25 percent). But then, those more endurance-oriented activities do not build muscle or strength the way weight training does.

As far as calorie burning is concerned, weight training—if it's done in "circuit" fashion (see note)—expends somewhere between six and nine calories a minute. That's roughly the equivalent of jogging at a 12-minute-per-mile pace, cycling at 11.5 miles per hour, or engaging in a vigorous game of volleyball or tennis. "An average man of 175 pounds could expect to lose approximately one-third of a pound of fat a month if he exercised using circuit weight training three days a week," Drs. Gettman and Pollock report.

So, according to those doctors, the bottom line on lifting weights to lose weight is: "Circuit weight training can be used as a weight-control program, although compared with aerobic training programs, the change in total body weight may not be as apparent, because the increases in lean body weight (muscle) and the losses in body fat may offset each other."

And as for cardiovascular purposes, "circuit weight training should not be considered an adequate aerobic program, but should include supplemental aerobic activity for optimal development of cardiorespiratory fitness," Drs. Gettman and Pollock note.

They do point out, however, that circuit training can be just what the doctor ordered for runners to keep fit while nursing an injury. "Two studies showed that subjects who reduced their jogging mileage by as much as 50 percent still maintained their cardiovascular endurance for 5 to 15 weeks" by training with weights, they said.

Why?

Because "once fitness is attained, it takes less effort to maintain."

Now *there's* good news.

NOTE: Circuit weight training has been defined by Drs. Gettman and Pollock as consisting of "two or three circuits of ten exercises designed so that the total workout time is between 25 and 30 minutes. These circuits generally consist of 10 to 15 repetitions per set at approximately 50 percent of maximum strength per exercise and 15 to 30 seconds rest between sets."

Q/ Is it bad to hold back a sneeze?

A/ A sneeze is a reflex action initiated by an irritation to the membranes lining the nose, and whether the irritation is caused by a particle of dust or the tickling sensation sometimes indicative of an oncoming cold, it's best to let it run its course. By suppressing a sneeze through shallow breathing, you only postpone it. And by letting the explosion happen (but keeping it to yourself by closing your mouth or pinching your nose), you can create enough pressure to cause a nosebleed—or, if you've got a cold, drive germs backward into the sinuses and lungs.

The best thing to do is let it go—but with restraint, and into a handkerchief. Broadcasting a sneeze at full blast in a car of an average-sized commuter train can spread tiny germ-infested droplets of vapor throughout most of the compartment—and that's the way diseases such as mumps, measles, whooping cough, influenza, and the common cold have their uncanny knack of "getting around."

Q/ What causes a hangover?

A/ Beer, scotch, gin, bourbon, wine, vodka, and something my brother once made out of apple cider. What remains in doubt is *how*.

Your headache, it's felt, is a result of swollen arteries in your brain. Your nausea, doctors seem to agree, is due to irritated membranes lining your gastrointestinal tract. And as for that inexorable thirst, that's your body's water table trying to get back what your night of whoopy saw fit to replace with cheap scotch. Anything else bothering you is the result of simple fatigue.

For the head, you can take aspirin; the stomach, a mild antacid or milk; and the thirst, anything *but* some more of the hair of that dog—it only postpones the inevitable.

Does it make a difference *what* you drink? Not as much as how much, but certain beverages do have more toxic substances—called congeners—than others, and hangovers actually have been induced by these "on the rocks" alone. Bourbon contains the most, followed by pure malt scotch, brandy and rum, blended scotch, vodka, and gin. White wine is low. Red wine falls somewhere between bourbon and scotch.

Finally, there's the psychological factor. If you drink when you're depressed or feeling guilty, says Morris Chafetz, M.D., former director of the National Institute on Alcohol Abuse and Alcoholism, you're going to pay for it. The moral is to imbibe without remorse, and only when you're relaxed —and happy.

Q/ How does squash stack up as aerobic (cardiovascular) exercise?

A/ According to a study done recently by David L. Montgomery, Ph.D., squash (and racquetball, if played with similar intensity) appears to be every bit as aerobic as running. Dr. Montgomery measured the heart rates of ten men who were both recreational runners and squash players. And he found that the *average* heart rates of those men as they played squash came very close to their average heart rates as they ran. Their heart rates averaged 173 beats per minute during a 45-minute running session (which came to an average of 84 percent of their maximum) as compared to 167 beats per minute (80 percent of maximum) for the 45 minutes that they played squash. Thus, "based on mean heart rate and percent intensity, running and squash produced similar responses," Dr. Montgomery said.

It's important to note, however, that the ball was in play in Dr. Montgomery's studies for an average of 52 percent of total time played. And the average duration of a rally was 7.7 seconds. So if your idea of a game of squash is a flashy serve against a not-so-flashy opponent, you may *not* be getting the cardiovascular workout that you would by running. It's important that players be of "equal ability and fitness level," Dr. Montgomery said. The better you are, in fact, the better the workout you're apt to be getting. For what Dr. Montgomery calls "A-level" players, studies have shown that the ball stays in play an admirably exhausting 69 percent of the time (*Physician and Sportsmedicine*, April, 1981).

Q/ Is it true that vasectomies can increase risks of heart disease?

A/ The jury on that question is still out. As stated in the British medical journal *Lancet* (November 17, 1979), "In short term at least, there is no clinical evidence that vasectomy is harmful in man. However, the possibility of rare or long-term effects cannot yet be ruled out."

Why?

A recently published study by Thomas Clarkson, D.V.M., of the Bowman Gray School of Medicine, and Nancy Alexander, Ph.D., of the Oregon Regional Primate Research Center, revealed that monkeys vasectomized 9 to 14 years prior to the study developed fatty deposits in several major blood vessels at rates greater than monkeys that had not been vasectomized. Blood tests showed why: The monkeys had developed antibodies to sperm (or their breakdown products) that had leaked into their bloodstreams as a result of not having their normal place to go. (Vasectomy, remember, ties off the vas deferens, or sperm duct.) The scientists theorized that this, in turn, was creating coagulation as antibodies would latch onto these unknown invaders, cause damage to the artery walls, and allow for more rapid development of atherosclerosis (hardening of the arteries) (*Journal of Clinical Investigation,* January, 1980).

Whether or not that happens in humans, however, is not yet known. Several studies have shown that vasectomized men do develop antibodies to their sperm. But thus far no studies done with humans (and there are several underway) have revealed any connection to atherosclerosis.

The question is important enough, however, for the National Institutes of Health to have funded three massive studies to look into the issue of vasectomy and its relation to cardiovascular disease.

"Results from these research efforts, though, are not likely to be in for another three to five years," Thomas Wegmann, Ph.D., an immunologist from the University of Alberta, told us. He advised anyone considering a vasectomy to hold off until more is known.

Q/ Does the ability to build muscle diminish with age?

A/ Yes, but not as drastically as your own withering biceps might suggest. "Substantial gains" can be made at "nearly any age," the owner of Expo Fitness Centers, Roger Servin, told us. (A runner-up in Mr. World body-building competition at age 43, Servin now is in peak form, at 50, to try again in the masters division of the Mr. America competition.) "Many of the best body builders in the business—Boyer Coe, for example—don't even reach their peak until about 40," Mr. Servin believes. "It takes that long in some cases to perfect the techniques that make a champion."

"Techniques" is a key word in Mr. Servin's assessment. Because laboratory studies have shown that while weight training may not produce as much muscle *growth* in older people, it *does* produce as much strength (see graph). The reason appears to be that the older we get, the better we become at learning to activate the nerves that make muscle fibers contract. (In one study which measured maximal grip strengths in 100 men who did similar work in a machine shop, no differences were found to exist even though the men ranged in age from 22 to 62.) "These data suggest that . . . [strength] losses with age may be due largely to disuse phenomena rather than a true aging effect," Herbert A. deVries, Ph.D., remarked on the study.

And that's encouraging on several accounts. First, it means there's no reason we shouldn't be able to beat our kids in arm wrestling right up until we retire; and second, it means that with a little bit of work, we can substantially put the brakes on the middle-age tendency to get fat. Because, as Dr. deVries explained, it is a loss in muscle tone that appears to be responsible for the slowing down of our metabolisms, and hence the tendency to gain weight (in the form of fat) as we age.

Muscle Changes from Weight Training

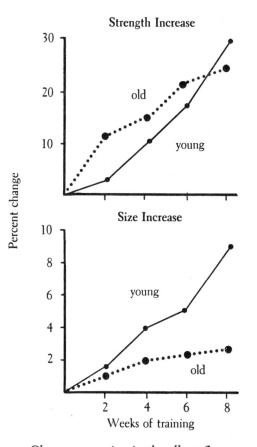

Changes occurring in the elbow flexor muscles of young and old men during weight training.

SOURCE: Adapted from and reprinted by permission of *Journal of Gerontology* (vol. 35, no. 5, 1980).

Q/ How do diet pills work and are they dangerous?

A/ Most work on a part of the brain that controls the appetite, and yes, they can be dangerous.

The active ingredient in the most popular brands being sold is phenyl-propanolamine, a laboratory-produced compound that reduces appetite by affecting the hypothalamus (the part of the brain that controls appetite), the taste buds, and the sense of smell.

As for the appetite-controlling chewing gums, most of these contain benzocaine, another laboratory-produced compound (also found in cough syrups) that works in a slightly different way: as a topical anesthetic that puts to sleep the taste buds on the tongue (idea being that no one is going to eat a lot of *anything* that he can't taste). Many of the phenylpropanolamine products also contain caffeine to give diet-induced fatigue.

Side effects? If used according to package instructions, the phenyl-propanolamine products say they can cause nothing more serious than headaches, dry mouth, and cramps. Dizziness or heart palpitations, they warn, can occur in some people, in which case their use should be discontinued. (A single dose of one especially strong phenylpropanolamine product sold in Australia, however, was found to raise blood pressure to dangerously high levels even in normal, healthy volunteers.)

In light of these dangers, the FDA recommends taking no more than 75 milligrams of phenylpropanolamine in any 24-hour period. Phenyl-propanolamine should not be taken *at all* by anyone with high blood pressure, diabetes, or disease of the heart, kidney, or thyroid; by pregnant or nursing women; by anyone under the age of 18; or by anyone taking medication for depression.

Should you try diet pills? We think not, for even though they may work for a while in some cases, the following case, as related by Edwin Bayrd in his book *The Thin Game* (Newsweek Books, 1978), serves as a fitting example of their overall worth: "The young woman managed to lose more than 50 pounds . . . on her . . . 13 pills a day. That she later gained all 50 back —plus 20 more she had not been carrying before she began her ill-advised diet—is a tragic testimony to the net effect of any diet that does not insist on a fundamental restructuring of existing eating habits and sound nutritional reeducation."

Q/ Why can some people drink more than others?

A/ Because they work at it. Body weight and metabolism come into play less than a lot of people think; being able to hold one's liquor, unfortunately, is mainly just a matter of practice.

Tolerance to alcohol develops along two fronts. One is physical: The liver gradually increases its ability to remove alcohol from the blood.

The other aspect of tolerance is mental, and it's here where people can get into trouble. If the brain were set up to get used to the effects of alcohol at the same rate as the body, there'd be no problem. But it isn't. Psychological tolerance beats physical tolerance to the punch, with the result being that the heavy drinker in many cases is actually drunker physically than he thinks. And so who smacks up his car on the way home from your party? The guy who "seemed" so sober. He thought he was, too.

Tolerance to alcohol *can* be reversed, but only by cutting down on intake, or contracting liver disease, as we've mentioned. If you're no longer getting the lift you used to from your before-dinner cocktail, it could be time to slow down.

Q/ Can stress cause gray hair?

A/ "It can be a factor," Irwin I. Lubowe, M.D., a dermatologist and author of numerous skin and hair care books told us. Hair turns gray—or white, actually—due to a lack of pigment (melanin) produced by the cortex of the hair shaft. That is most directly related to aging, but environmental factors —stress and diet—also can come into play.

"There have been extreme cases in wartime situations, for example," Dr. Lubowe told us, "where melanin secretions have stopped in direct response to extreme emotional duress." (That, of course, would not cause hair to whiten at the moment, but the effects *would* begin to show as the new colorless hairs grew out.)

Nutrition is another potential contributor—both pro and con. "Laboratory tests with black rats have shown that feeding them a diet deficient in the B vitamins turned their hair white," reports Philip Kingsley in the *Complete Hair Book* (Fred Jordan/Grosset and Dunlap, 1979). "On reintroducing vitamin B, the hair regained its color."

Dr. Lubowe told us he has had some success in both preventing and treating whitened hair by prescribing 500 milligrams each of pantothenic acid and PABA (para-aminobenzoic acid) twice daily for about six months. Kingsley has had luck with "large doses of vitamin B, particularly in the form of brewer's yeast and defatted liver extract."

In light of Dr. Lubowe's war stories, it wouldn't hurt also to learn how to relax. And if *that* doesn't work, wear your white proudly, as a sign of experience.

Q/ Is it healthful to drink wine with meals?

A/ It can be, provided you take into consideration the additional calories that wine supplies (see table on cocktails and their calories, in chapter 4). Wine, besides having its own modest amounts of vitamins and minerals, has been shown to enhance the absorption of calcium, phosphorus, magnesium, iron, and zinc. And wine also may allay some of the ill effects of a cholesterol-rich diet, as evidenced by experiments with rats and hamsters in which "the increase in liver fat and cholesterol and serum cholesterol [after eating cholesterol-rich foods] was significantly less in the wine-fed group than in groups fed an alcohol solution or water" (*Professional Nutritionist,* Summer, 1981).

As for appetite control, wine appears to be a kind of equalizer. For obese people, it can reduce appetite and lessen anxieties about eating (a tranquilizing effect some people attribute to properties in wine other than its alcohol). For people with depressed appetites, however, wine seems to stimulate the appetite, both by activating gastric functions and—again—by alleviating stress. So . . .

Even though wine's calories could be considered relatively empty from a nutritional standpoint, they would seem capable of offering more benefits (in moderation, of course) than the calories in many condiments (i.e., butter, margarine, salad dressings, and sugar). Better a "yes, please" to the wine steward, in other words, than to the fellow passing around the sour cream.

INDEX

A

B